STREA
ICE

by John McKelvie

All rights reserved, no part of this publication may be reproduced by any means, electronic, mechanical, or photocopying, documentary, film, or otherwise without prior permission of the publisher.

Published by:
Chipmukapublishing
PO Box 6872
Brentwood
Essex
CM13 1ZT
United Kingdom

http://www.chipmunkapublishing.com

Copyright © 2007 John McKelvie

It goes without saying that names have been changed. Except Streatham and Brixton and places.

4

STREATHAM ICE

EDUCATION

I saw him at the enrolling. There were hordes of us in the gymnasium, alphabetically divided. You could see him from the back even though he'd hacked his little red dreads off. McEwan. Smoking against the rules. Good boy.

He looked round once, didn't see me of course, wouldn't recognise me anyway, being dressed up, different from school. I felt nervous. Everyone else was screaming and jerking about like party kids. I knew some of them. But McEwan was on his own, like me. A bottle sticking out his pocket.

He swanked up to the table where the officials sat. His turn to enrol. He landed the old girl, shook her hand and made her smile. A few questions, then suddenly a fuss. He hadn't brought his photographs. You were supposed to have two. He didn't have one. He couldn't enrol.
"Please", said McEwan like a spoilt brat.
"Sorry. No", said the old girl, very final.
They stared at each other. Then he pulled the gun.

Someone screamed. Enrolling stopped. Danger in the gymnasium. He turned to the audience, gun flat against his chest. Everyone moved back.
"I'm not just a pretty face. Whatever she thinks. I've got feelings too, you know, feelings - "

He couldn't go on, choked. I wanted to clap, show him I cared, but I kept quiet. I trusted him. The woman leaned forward being brave. She wasn't stupid. The gun was see-through green.

"Mr McEwan", she said calmly. "Put your water pistol away and go and get your photographs at the post office. Then you can enrol. And, if I may say so, your joke is in particularly bad taste given the current climate of gun crime in this borough."

Oooooh, went the crowd.

He looked at her, poked the gun in his ear and closed his eyes.

"All I wanted was an education," he said.

He squeezed the trigger. Splash. He staggered off, ear dripping.

Someone jeered, the gymnasium breathed, and the queue jerked on, excited. Enrolling continued. McEwan was left alone. Noone dared touch him. He took out the Smirnoff and put it back again, empty.

"Bloody nutter", said a cheeky Asian boy in front, and his friends choked themselves. McEwan turned to them, hands out, urgent. They stepped back.

"Here we stand, bruvvers, waiting to be educated, while the illiterate racist mobs of Britain are on the streets threatening your mothers, your sisters, your freeDUM. And all she -" he jabbed his finger at the brave lady "- all she goes on about is f-f-fucking p-p-passport photos." He looked up at the roof and cried: "Dear God, give us da peace."

Some applause for that. The boys laughed. He reached for his gun and they jumped. They didn't trust him. He smiled, slotted his dark specs on and left, acting blind, guided with care by the matey college porter who had convinced me and me Mum when we visited that Lambeth College sure is coming up in the world. Most of the other kids at school went to Wandsworth or Richmond or Wimbledon for A levels, anywhere but Lambeth, but what did they know? Basically, I was sick of school and GCSEs and being treated like a brat and no way was I going to travel miles just to pass more exams.

McEwan hadn't seen me yet, but he would. I was confident. Maybe he never got the photos. Maybe he never enrolled. I dunno. I'd got mine that morning at Sainsbury's, came out looking like a Bash Street Kid. Four times. The future looked good.

BOYS

By the third day we'd met. I saw him in the canteen, alone, long black scarf wound round tight, his new red hair slicked back, unlit fag in mouth, new books on table, sunburnt face gone freckly, blue eyes staring. The wild boy look. I went over.

"Allo. Remember me?"
It took him long enough. We'd not been friends at school, just smokers. He pulled that stupid smile.
"Yeah. Course. Good to see you. Sit down, mate."
"I'm Alex," I said, to help him. "How are you?"
"I'm good. Very good, Alex. And I am – " pause for effect " – McEwan."
He always gushed in those days. And he told me about his hot holiday in Spain, specially pleased at the Moroccan draw he'd sneaked home in the family foot pump.
"Later," he said tapping his breast pocket. "But first I'd like to buy you a drink. A Spanish special. To celebrate our reunion."
That was a joke. Still, it was a very promising start.

I phoned me Mum and told her I'd met an old mate. That's nice love, she said, pleased I was fitting in.

I followed him leaping downstairs to the Basement Tapas Bar in a Clapham side street. McEwan gave me his books and went off waving at the small barman. He came back with two tall glasses of golden syrup packed with ice. And a plate of fish on toast.

"To the future".
"To Lambeth College."
"Our further education"
We had two more large ones. With eggs and olives and more toast. We were getting along nicely.
"I remember you," he said, like he'd just remembered. "You gave me two cigs before a GCSE. I failed em all."
I didn't believe him.

"Listen to this".
He had a paper, the local horror stories. He read it out, choking.
"59 years old school teacher Audrey Harris was the victim of a terror campaign waged by two ex-pupils of her class at Sunnyside Primary School, SW16. The boys, aged eleven and twelve -"
"Fucking toddlers."
"- took their revenge on Miss Harris for her old-fashioned teaching methods. Their gruesome acts included posting live frogs through her letter-box, fatally frothing her fishpond with detergent and yelling suddenly behind her in the street, causing her to jump and twist her ankle."
McEwan creased up. I carried on.
"The two boys were caught red-handed climbing out of Miss Harris' back garden carrying spray-paint cans having graffiti'd her bird bath. Silver-haired Miss Harris is due to retire at the end of this

school year. After 32 years of service, she will be sad to leave, but she is critical of today's standards of behaviour. She said - "
McEwan snatched it back. In a high-pitched teacher screech:
"I follow simple rules based on what's good and bad, right and wrong. Some children and, I'm sad to say, their parents, don't know the difference any more".
He threw the paper away.
"Poor old girl".
"No respect".
"Bet she's a right old cow though".
"And boys - you know - will be BOYS."
"Yeah."
We leapt up the basement steps into the warm, fumy street. McEwan's books were still in the bar but he didn't go back. We charged into the sunset on Clapham Common.

"The churchyard," he said. "Best place to smoke."
An old stinker was wobbling around the Angel of Temperance monument, a Red Stripe sticking out his coat pocket. I was going to miss him out but McEwan slowed down.
"Scuze me, sir," said the stinker, putting his hand out.
"Yes, sir?" said McEwan. "What's the problem?"
The man was surprised.
"I got no money. Fra cup of tea."
"Here, treat yourself, mate. Have a large one."
McEwan gave him a couple of quid, patted him on the shoulder and left him shocked.

"They don't ask for much. And remember, Alex, it's the simple things in life that count. Good and bad and aaaagh - "

He was rattling the railings and screaming, like a lunatic. Then we were over and into the graveyard, leaping along the crazy paving.

And so it happened, in the churchyard, amongst the graves, getting dark, we smoked and relaxed. No legs. Free at last. I couldn't move.

The church spire pointed towards heaven. We stood up to get closer. Then we lay down for the gravity. And then McEwan knelt and prayed.

"O sacred spire up in the sky
So tall and straight and very high
We come to you -
me mate Alex here and I - "

He collapsed. I laughed at him laughing, laughed at nothing, laughed up all my tapas on the gravel-chip path. God I was sick. Orrible, gravely sick.

"Bad mix," I explained to my mother who said I was the colour of an old dishcloth. She never really disapproved, me Mum, just made me feel stupid.

MOTHER

Me Mum, who I love, works long hours with troubled kids, an experienced nurse. She met my dad when she was training and he was a hospital-porter student-drop-out punk-rebel. They got married fast, for fun and a big party. How was she to know that, two years later, when I was a babe in arms and he was out of his head, he'd do his famous fourth floor balcony balancing trick and, for the last time, fall off? Dead.

We live in Streatham Hill, London Borough of Lambeth. Next to Brixton on the road to Brighton, as me Mum says. She's lived around here since she was a student nurse and never moved, what with Brixton market, her yoga man and veggie caff, not to mention the Italian on the High Road where Elvis sings at weekends.

She lives a quiet life now, doesn't go out much - for a smashing time, that is - just a meal or movie with her main friend Jane. And she visits the old couple downstairs for deaf chat and tea and they tell her Streatham ain't what it used to be, what wiv all them asylum people here, darlin. And she just listens, she's kind, she gets upset, then she comes back and tells me:
"Mary thinks they send refugees here from Brixton. I tell her, Brixton's only down the road, Mary. Oh I know darlin, she says, but it's a different world down there."

Her own parents live in Yorkshire. We sometimes go there for a holiday but they never visit us, Grannie being anxious and cold and Granpa being embarrassing.

As I got older, she worked more and more hours with the troubled kids. Sometimes she'd tell me about them going mad. I didn't get it, her getting up really early in the morning just to go there and get cussed all day. She went to the yoga man to be calm.

We used to do a lot together when I was younger. Shows and movies, museums and shops. She loved mad old clothes. And dancing. She used to go to a salsa class at the Starlight Studios down the High Road with a plumber called Stuart. We went to Amsterdam with him when I was ten and went crazy on bikes. Stuart bought some spliffs in a cafe and they must have got wasted after I'd gone to bed. They were still giggling at breakfast.

She took me to the Ice Rink once when I was 7 or 8, like all Streatham kids do. Neither of us could skate. We held hands and ended up in a heap. At first it was funny then some girls from my school sailed past us like the Olympics and laughed at me splat out on the ice with me Mum, twice. I hated that.
"You'll learn, love," she said, gagging her giggles.
"Don't want to," I said, hurt and humiliated.
That was one of the worst moments of my life. I'd failed the Streatham ice test. I refused to go

again, of course, even on the most bored days. Too proud, she'd say, you're just too proud.

But don't worry, I'm not a complete nan. I started skateboarding at the Clapham paddling pool when I was 12. Then Stockwell Park where there were no Streatham schoolgirls to see me lurking on the edge. Me Mum took me there the first couple of times and went off and left me to survive. The boys there were OK but not friends. I saw Mum sneaking a look once, checking like I was a kid, and I went on at her till she let me go by myself. When I had my bike snatched, I ran home and never went back. Ex skate punk.

She still got nervous about me of course, especially when I got jacked twice on the High Road in year 10. First time, two boys borrowed my brand new phone. Second time, some rude boys smacked me and another boy round the face for cheeking them, which we hadn't. Mum was badly angry and upset. She was convinced I'd get knifed next. She made me go to the police who went yeah there's a couple of gangs making trouble in Streatham. Well what are you doing about them then? she shouts and bangs the desk, then she apologised and said she was all upset, being a mother, but she knows it's not just the police's problem, she works with troubled kids herself and knows the community has to deal with it.

"Community?" went the copper, sarcastic. "What's that, madam? Ha ha."

"Yes," said me Mum, very definite. "The community. You, me, the schools, the parents, the neighbours. I mean, what about all the gun crime round here? Alex could get <u>shot</u>, Officer."

"As long as your boy keeps clear of Jamaican crack dealers, he should be alright, madam," said the policeman, reassuring.

"So just be careful who you buy your drugs from, love." Mum winked at me.

The copper didn't laugh and I blushed. She could be like that - make you embarrassed and make you proud.

I lost my nerve, didn't go out much, and me Mum worried I was getting anti-social, staying in and watching crap TV. She started driving me places and collecting me, then decided that life was hard and I had to get used to it, she couldn't protect me forever. She was full of good advice. She said:

"Being a boy in London is tough, so you've got to be smart. Don't go upstairs on the bus. Avoid eye contact. Get a girlfriend. Use a condom. No knives. Hand over the cash. And run fast." She held my hands and looked deep in my eyes. "Be proud, my son, but watch it, alright?"

"Thanks Mum."

A good person, me Mum, tough in her own way, but she was soft on me. She wanted me to be strong, make friends and take care, love. Sometimes her fussing and worrying got on my nerves and I'd scream at her. I could do that with her. And she could scream at me too, then she'd always come and say sorry love, but I generally didn't. She says I've got my dad's dark irresistible eyes. And his pride. He always had to win.

"Just watch it, Alex," she said.

MAKING FRIENDS

Me and McEwan started going into town for the bars and the buzz and it was, well, better than Streatham. I thought he'd been loads of times before, but he probably hadn't. I knew more about street life than him, I read the gutter press. But he had the nerve and somehow I got it too.

"If you like it, lift it," he said, the big anarchist. "Global economy, global ownership."
I hated him lifting at first. We went into Borders and he walked out with a pile of books on his head. I felt sick, till I did it too - magazines and deodorants at first - and got a deep thrill. Difference was, he lifted in public, and I did it as secretly as possible.

We dressed up for town, cheap and loose, big on army surplus. McEwan nicked me a black cap, like his. My time had come. McEwan acted like he owned the place, swanking in and out, talking to people, laughing loud, getting looks and getting cussed. He picked up tourists and gave them the wrong directions. He hated Americans most because of the Indians and MacDonald's and everything. And we both hated football shirts. They had nothing we wanted. I support Crystal Palace cos me Mum says my Dad did so she does and I do, but I never go. McEwan said football fucks, but I decided Palace didn't count cos they never do much.

Lounging under Nelson, gurgling in his vodka and cafe freddo louder than Trafalgar Square, he spied a statue they painted last May Day.

"Major General Sir Henry Havelock of the British Empire, Alex. Destroyed three Indian armies. Painted green on May Day.... Hey, look at *her*. Er excuse me, senorita. You like young Englishman?"

We got a look, a smile if we were lucky. McEwan loved dark shiny girls. I liked anything. And there were millions of them in town, swinging Mango bags and swaying their bums left right and centre. Oh yeah. Lots of queer boys too, marking us, specially in Soho. But we liked girls. Especially girls who didn't like us.

We drank cheap beverages in fashionable places, on the watch, saving cash for fags and drugs. We nicked nice drinks and leftovers in busy bars and cool caffs. Noone notices and if they do you just go sorry mate, bad mistake. I drink anything, except cider which makes me edgy and whiskey which makes me sick.

There was a wrinkled old Jamaican singer in one Soho bar, with gold teeth and a white mac, who always remembered McEwan. He mumbled songs with feeling for us and McEwan always bought him a big rum for his trouble. He used to live in a hostel up there. Got too fancy round here for me now, he said. Awful fancy, he said with spit.

"Yeah, far too fucking fancy", we spat too.

The middle of London's like one big playtime, all day and all night. You stand still in Leicester Square and you spin. You get drink, draw and deals, and you make new friends from across da whole wide world. Fun time, big time, man!

But *we* knew where to go for <u>real</u> low class entertainment. Nightspot, near the river, claustrophobic and cheap, for kids in the know. We were members for life. Just a damp cellar, low on special effects and strong on danger signs. Shocking slideshow on wet black walls and drum and bass that took your pulse. *Bad boys ina London, rude boys ina Brixton. Bad boys ina London, rude boys ina Kingston.* Jamaica. The cops dawnraided it. The neighbours wanted it bombed. They blamed the foreign DJs and the wide choice of drugs. For us kids it was just a nice place to make friends.

Like Lucy one night. She was standing on her own. Purple lips, short sharp black hair, floppy fringe. Bit of a Goth but I liked her. I stopped casually beside her, accidentally touched.
"Allo."
She stared at me. She was on something pretty soul-destroying. Must get some.
"Allo I'm Alex." I tried again.
She giggled.
"I'm Lucille. L-L-Lucy." She laughed dangerously, then hugged me like it really mattered and said, "You're a very, very nice boy." And choked again.

Then her boy arrived, wet from dancing. He smiled, put his arms around her and rocked her, calmed her down. A good boy.

"Thanks, mate," he said to me, like I'd been nursing her.

"No problem, mate."

"Rico," he introduced himself and shook hands. "Want anything, mate?"

A small deal of E's was struck and we lingered on, jerking about headless and screaming. He became our best seller. Almost a mate.

McEwan and I invented a big dance there designed to attract girls, involving loadsa straining and stomping. We made a good pair, him and me. He was tall and all over the place; I kept it tight. He was loud and I was quiet. He had a pierced eyebrow; not me, mate. But did we attract girls and make loads of new friends? Course not. So what? Thank God for the Spot. It closed a few weeks later.

It was NightSpot where I first saw Karen whom I shall tell you about in a minute. She didn't notice me, of course. She never stopped dancing.

PRIDE

Me Mum could be dumb but she could also be wise. She said:
"You've grown up with all the love and attention of one woman, no dad or brothers or sisters to share me with. So watch out, Alex. No one else thinks you're special like I do and you can get badly hurt with that pride of yours."
She didn't tell me what to do about it, of course. And if she had, I wouldn't have listened, would I, being so, so proud?

Respect was her philosophy, not pride. Respect for yourself, respect for others. She told me things about my dad to flash warning signs about his reckless pride, no self-respect.
"Sean always had to go one better, get drunker, louder, madder than anyone else. He had to be the one to walk along the balcony ledge. And of course he had to die first, didn't he? And that really put the lid on it. He won that one, no question."

Me being her only boy, her pride and joy, she didn't want me taking an early bath too, did she? Scuse the football reference but basically she wanted me safe and strong and respected, like a boy Beckham in Streatham. She respected him, even if he had no GCSEs.

She remembered how I used to hate school cos the teachers knew more than I did. And my fights with Rufus, my best mate at primary school.

"You hated it if Rufus beat you in a test, you wouldn't talk to him. Remember when his mother accosted me one day cos her Rufus was so upset you'd taken his best computer game and you told me you took it because he'd passed the entrance exam to that posh school and you didn't want to lose your best friend."

That's what I told me Mum anyway but I just nicked it really. I wanted his Super Mario Bros. I was gonna give it back, wasn't I? I liked Rufus a lot but I hated him after that. He was always telling his mum about me. Creep. He went to some smart school in Wandsworth and I didn't have a best mate again till McEwan. I had other mates and girls at senior school and had a laugh, course I did, but noone special. Best mates squeal and do you in.

Then there were the street attacks. I hated the bums who nicked my bike and phone. There's nothing you can do. They boss it, like older kids do when you start school. So basically I quit going out, my sad way of getting revenge by depriving them of the opportunity to do me, not that they'd exactly notice my absence.

I went to a couple of Ki-Aikido classes, self-defence for me Mum's nerves, but it was crap and going up the other end of Streatham on a Monday night was dangerous in itself. So I just stayed in and fantasised about <u>really</u> defending myself. Like carrying a gun and scaring them. So when they stop me, push me and pull me for me valuables, I go: I got nuffin mate, but I got <u>this</u>. And out comes my little Baby Beretta like a real neat death threat, and they run and I've won. I don't think so.

Pride. It's what got me into a bit of a fix later on, but we'll come to that, cos this is my little tale of a bruvver's pride, a lover's pride and a muvver's pride. Clever, eh? It's about how me, Alex, got hurt and defended my pride. Which basically you've gotta do, haven't you? It's the least you can do. Respect is for later, Mum. OK?

Cos right now I gotta tell you about Karen.

SEX AND GAMBLING IN BRIXTON

Friday night, The Trinity Arms, backstreets of Brixton, no cool styling, just a plain boozer in wood and mirrors. The usual six o'clock mix of dolls and dealers, tattoo artists and builders in shorts, muttering old girls and wounded soldiers, all laughing at each other.

McEwan's in his tight childhood grey hoodie with TAWT in big red marker on the back. Me in black. I wanted to look right, more confident about my sex appeal nowadays, specially with McEwan there. Not that he was so great, just that, like I said, he had nerve.

A dull evening so far. Two dangerous drinks and still no thrills. McEwan starts the intros with two neat personal assistants standing nearby. They swallow their drinks and go up in smoke. Not a look, not a cuss.
"Piss off", he moans to the vacant space.
"Their loss," I say.
"Yeah." He thrusts his fist up.

At the bar the thinnest man in Brixton is rolling his fags for the night. Three nervous breakdowns have undone their necks and are roaring at every line. McEwan goes to the bar and gets involved with three more PA's who start touching up his long black hairy scarf. He slips off the scarf and winds it round one of their necks. She loves it. He waves me over. Then one of the slack-tie nervous breakdowns puts his nose in -

"Got a problem, mate?" He's with the PA's.

"Nothing pressing", says McEwan.

"Well that's alright then, isn't it? You alright, Tina?"

"Course I'm alright," says Tina. "We're having a laugh, aren't we love? OK, Jason?"

Jason scans the funny boy. Then McEwan says so politely:

"I'm sorry, I hadn't realised that you were responsible for these charming ladies, sir."

"Is he taking the piss?" says Jason.

"You dummy. He's just a kid. He's lovely," says Tina.

"Funny boy, are we?" Jason smiles at McEwan, uncertain.

"Not me, sir." McEwan bows, turns and withdraws, flicking V-signs that Jason can't see, big grin on his face, twitching his TAWT at Jason.

"Fuck", he says. "We were getting along so sweet too, Tina and me. Shame."

"Sorry, love," says one of the PA's as she goes past to the bog. "Jason's just a dickhead. Can't take competition. Especially from nice young boys."

"So kind", says McEwan.

What a charmer that boy could be.

You know how one thing always leads to another? McEwan and I get shouting about dickheads and global domination and McEwan's accusing MTV and MacDonald's and Microsoft of poisoning the food we eat, the air we breathe and the thoughts we think and I say you can't say that and this dickhead at the next table who's been earwigging us leans over and goes:

"Excuse me for butting in, guys, but don't you think that globalisation is in the eye of the beholder? Your dreaded global economy could equally be my brotherhood of man or the Rough Guide to World Music or - "

What? This bum is with the girl I'd seen dancing at NightSpot. Fuck! Sounds too clever by half to me, but McEwan finds him funny. Anything you mention, he has a line about it. He's got McEwan and the girl chuckling every time. I like her. I like her clothes and her laugh. A lot. This is KAREN. And he's Ian, a large maths lecturer, far too old for her, it's obvious. A smart arse and big mouth. Listen. He's telling us how he gets a sexual kick doing sums with people on the net and climbing Welsh mountains. He talks about sex alot, so he can impress bashful boys like me and McEwan. McEwan says, sensitive and confidential:

"I think sex is a very personal matter and prefer to keep it to myself. Keep sex off our mountain sides, I say."

"Sounds like you just wank a lot", says Ian.

"Loads, but at least I do it in private."

"Touché."

They strike fists, like gangsta mates. Karen sticks a finger down her throat, disgusted. Boys eh? Oh yeah.

They like us, buy us drinks. And when the pub shuts they ask us back to Karen's flat up Brixton Hill for more blag and laughs. Yes! I'll come back, Karen, anything. She's living with her cousin and her cousin's partner, comes from Bath, doing a gap year as a bookstore café barrista, saving up to travel and get highly educated. Ian's a scouser. He has a home up there and a young family to whose open arms he sometimes returns. Bastard.

On Acre Lane, Ian crosses himself at a lamppost with some old bunches of flowers leaning on it.
"Some poor bugger got gunned down here last week," he says. "It was on the telly."
"Bloody ell," we go, looking for the signs.
"Brixton," says Ian, like that explained everything.

Karen's cousin Celia and her Chinese boyfriend Ho have a flat with style. They giggle and smile a lot and give us rum and smoke with Basement Jax. I'm watching Karen. McEwan says anyone for dice? and noone says no. He pulls out three dice and shows them a game he'd learnt in Spain, a boring and dangerous game called Trio, with a religious meaning. God. McEwan loved it. He clears a space on the floor and issues instructions.
"It's simple. You throw all the dice and divide the total by three. Only exact divisions' count and the lowest division wins. A flush beats a run and a run beats a mixed throw."
"And how do you bet?" Ian asks, hooked.
"Right," says McEwan and smiles threateningly. "You stake what you throw, yeah? So if you throw

three sixes, you stake 18. And the lowest division by three wins. So the more you throw, the more you have to stake and the more you lose. And the less you throw, the less you have to stake, the less you lose and of course, ladies and gentlemen, the more you win. So three ones is the answer to life itself."

"You what?" says Celia. "I didn't follow any of that."

"Ignore her," says Ho. "She can't count straight."

She throws a cushion at him and knocks the end off the spliff, burning a hole in his cool white trousers. He chucks it back, narked.

"Course Chinese boys gamble on anything, don't you darling?"

"No racial stereotypes please," says Ian. "All men gamble. Let's go."

He and Ho get on their knees with McEwan, keen to gamble, like all men do. I stay in my big chair. Karen stretches out on the sofa and yawns loudly. I stare. It's a fantastic sexy yawn.

"So why don't women gamble?" asks Celia, sweet and innocently.

"Because they represent safety not risk," says Ian, old and wisely. "Men are the risk-takers."

"Kak," goes Karen, loud and risky suddenly. "Women have better things to do with their time than go gambling, that's all. Ever been in a bookies? It's full of sad men stressing themselves so they feel something. Risk-takers? Wankers."

I'm staring at Karen thinking fuck!

Ian, of course, big guy, wins the dice game and big-heartedly donates all his winnings to their Friends of the Earth plastic globe, sits back against Karen's legs and she strokes his head and shoulders. I hated that. Then he tells us his story about dice.

"In my disturbed youth," he says, "I decided to let the dice dictate my life, like the guy in the book. What's his name? Shit. Anyway, I was ruled by random options. Like I robbed a launderette once but all the money was in the washing machines. Then I had to seduce my Physics teacher's wife. That was the best throw. Lovely lady. Then one day the dice told me to grow up and start making my own fucking decisions."

Ha ha ha. I don't think so.

Time to go home.

"So what's the difference between Streatham and Brixton?" Karen asks, being new to the area.

"You don't need a gun in Streatham," says Ian, cynical.

"Shut-up," Karen tells him. "You just hate Brixton."

Ian acts innocent. I believe her.

"Well. Streatham's a very fine place," gushes McEwan then dries up. "Er, isn't it, Alex?"

"Oh yes, mate," I help him out. "Not exactly cool but then it ain't really cool to live somewhere really cool, is it? Streatham is er real. Nowamin?"

"Er no," they all go.

"Well. Clapham's cool but – you know – " I explain. "And Brixton ain't just cool, it's more well completely crazy man. Yeah?"

"You what?" they scream like I'm talking crap.
Then McEwan gets dramatic.

"Streatham's got the longest loudest high road on earth and a wild and windy common where big dogs howl at the moon - " he howls " - and, and - a sparkling ice rink for – for our fun-loving youth."

"Sounds a very er happy place," says Karen.

"It's why we smile so much," I explain.

"No tube though," says Ho.

"And no Madonna one-nighters," screams Celia.

"Who wants her?" McEwan dumps Madonna.

"And what about Brixton's unique cultural fusion?" asks Ho.

"You mean the heady racial synergy of Coldharbour Lane?" checks Ian, for effect.

"That's right, smart arse," says Ho. "Streatham's way behind."

They wait for our response to the massive multicultural question, tense.

"You see, my friends, Streatham just ain't swamped -" says McEwan, thoughtful and daring, waiting and watching them wondering what the hell he's gonna say "- by rich young white kids who race up and down the Victoria Line and colonise the cafes and clubs and all the best houses in Brixton."

They look at each other, no answer.

"But Streatham's got no clubs and cafes to colonise," Celia cries and Ho whoops with relief.

"William Blake thought that Lambeth was the new Jerusalem," says Karen, raising the tone.

"That was before Streatham was built," says Ho.

"But don't forget -" McEwan begins but then blanks out.

"Yeah, don't forget -" I help out, struggling, "- that, that Naomi Campbell comes from Streatham."

That's a joke but somehow it sounds like I'm serious. There's a shocked silence. Then Ian shouts:

"The winner!" Yanking my hand up and down. "Naomi clinches it for Streatham!"

I felt dumb. Ian made me feel dumb. I hated him. He was funny and brainy and forty. He looked like a bear, but he had good stories. And sex with Karen. She was so cool. And I was too young. It was all so clear, it hurt.

Climbing slowly and painfully up Brixton Hill to boring sad Streatham, McEwan howling at the moon with his sick purple ski hat with earflaps on, I had Karen on my brain. Karen. I wanted her. I only wanted to be with Karen.

FURTHER EDUCATION

But I had to write two essays first. I kept dreaming off and seeing her, stretched out on that red sofa, yawning and laughing. The Russian Revolution was a real struggle and all I got was a C.

Six weeks at Lambeth College, and the authorities and McEwan already had a problem. He thought it was them, they thought it was him. Course, they had all the power and he just had an attitude and it didn't fit. Like when he embarrassed a Government and Politics teacher about her unnaturally long hair, then made a public apology in their next class when he called for the resignation of her head of department who had spoken to him, man to man, about respect and consideration for the woman's feelings. This man was a known sex-pest, said McEwan, and was in no position to lecture.

A lot of the kids avoided him. And he ignored them. But the canteen ladies loved him. He was a star. They touched his stubbly red hair and wobbly stud. He always had a kind word for them and they would ask after his cracked ribs which he only invented for attention. He took his favourite lady, Rose, a red one on her birthday, plucked from a florist's display. Nice boy McEwan.

Problem was he did no work at all and the teachers were issuing warnings, threatening to expose him as an A level fraud, which of course he was. He only took Government and Politics to sharpen up on urban terrorist techniques. But Mr Morrison, the cool and confident Head of English, took him under his wing and transferred him to his own set to ensure examination success. Let's get serious, Paul, he said to McEwan. (McEwan hated his first name. Paul made him feel small.)

Serious or not, McEwan never talked about college work and he had no plans for the future, as far as I could see. Me, I kept my options open. I didn't want to fail yet. Teachers and exams pissed me off alright but you don't have to think too hard and you get through it. But McEwan didn't see life like that. He couldn't compromise, he couldn't wait. He'd been excluded from St Joseph's Boys' College for badly letting the school down and came to our place to fuck his GCSEs up. Ours was the only school that would have him, being big and offering excellence for all, but they don't do A levels, so we both ended up at Lambeth College which, as the porter said, sure is going places. Lambeth College, by Clapham Common, is for kids from Brixton, Stockwell and Streatham, Lambeth kids all of us, just looking for survival and the best possible grades. Well most of us were.

McEwan never got the difference between fantasy and reality. Or pass and fail, for that matter. He didn't give a fuck. Sweet, sweet, sweet FE, he used to croon as we swung round the corridors looking for a class. He usually gave up.

KAREN

I kept thinking about her. Had to see her. Trouble was she already had mature man Ian and here's me just a boy, absolute beginner. Bloody ell.

I decided to front it and walked into the Waterstones cafe, casually, to see if she was working. She was. I bought a cappuccino. How are you? I said. She was sick of making cappuccino, sick of books and sick of men. I changed the subject.
"I saw you at NightSpot."
"Did you? I didn't see you."
"You didn't stop dancing. Look, can we meet up?"
"Why?" She was like that, getting to the heart.
"I'd like to see you."
She looked at me, different.
"OK," she said. "Do you dance?"
"All the time," I said and she twirled her hand in the air. Beautiful hands.
Yes!

We met at the Hobgoblin. She liked a bald blue-eyed barman there who never spoke. Powerful persona, she said. She drank Sol and smoked two of my cigs. Black jacket, brown eyes. She didn't have to wear much, just looked good. She said:
"How's your friend?"
"McEwan?"
"Yeah. Why's he called McEwan?"
"Cos he hates Paul. He's in trouble." I told her about his problems with the authorities.

"He thinks he's God's gift, doesn't he? He wants them to crucify him," she said, very wise and hitting the nail. "Tell him to make his own decisions."

"Hey, make your own decisions, mate. That's an order." I rehearsed the line and she stuck me in the ribs, like I was taking the piss. Fast action, sharp jab.

"Does he dance?"

"Yeah when he needs to. He wants me to go to a Brixton rap club with him."

"Radical," she said, sarcastic. "What's he know about rapping?"

"Not much, that's why he wants to learn. Very dedicated, you see. So lay off him, he's me mate."

"I liked him. Really. And his funny clothes."

They'd all screamed at his purple ski hat with the earflaps and I didn't much like them taking the piss. So I said:

"Very fussy about his clothes, he is. You wouldn't think so but he is. Very ethical too. No sweatshop kids' clothes for McEwan, oh no."

"Ethical." She laughed. Great mouth. "You mean worn. I'm the same. Like I check all the style mags then go and buy cheap charity shop kit."

"Ethical chic."

"Exactly."

She smiled. Yes! We understood each other.

She was desperately saving money from her coffee job to go travelling before university next year. She'd come from Bath to be in London, at the heart, on the pulse, lucky to get a room in

Brixton in her cousin's flat. Celia and her mate Ho spent all day working at home on computers.

"Something serious in websites," she said, "and it pays really well. Easyjets to European hotspots every weekend."

So excited, wasn't she, to be living in Brixton and the manic multi-culture, the clubs, the holy street choirs and the history. The royal visits of Mandela, Tyson and Madonna! She loved the mix. But she'd never heard of Streatham before.

"Streatham's just er lower-key," I said. "You can chill."

"Has it got a market? Brixton market is brilliant."

"I know. Me Mum goes there for her fancy greens."

"Cool."

"She kept me off school to see Nelson Mandela when he came here."

"Oh yeah?" She was well impressed. I'd never boasted about me Mum - or Nelson Mandela - to anyone before. It worked. Eyes wide. Brilliant eyes.

But the clubs were her real buzz. Dancing. Like that half-empty Tuesday night at NightSpot when I saw her jerking on and on, on her own. *I see you standing on the corner of the dance floor and the way you move you look so fine....* I didn't ask her about Ian. I didn't want to know. I wanted Karen to myself. And I wanted her to like me. A lot.

Had we got on good? Well tonight we ended up bobbing but no snogging in The Hobgoblin. She was class, man. And when she sprang off to her flat, like she did, she said thanks for the dance and I said, kind of joking, when can I see you again? And she just waved her arm in the air, halfway across screaming dangerous Brixton Hill. What?

MASS

Me Mum said I was looking dreamy, was it love or drugs? Mothers eh? She was relieved to hear I'd been out with a girl, girl company being safer than boys. And drugs, for that matter. She was pleased I was making friends in my new life at Lambeth College and getting out and about after a year of staying indoors and staying safe.

"No bother from the bad boys on the High Road then?" she enquired.

"My mate McEwan sees them off."

"How's he do that?" She was worried.

"Just smiles at them. He's a wild boy."

First time he came round to our flat he charmed me Mum, called her Mrs Alex and kissed her hand. She laughed, asked him about Lambeth College, and he said he was studying global capitalism and mass exploitation so he could fight for the poor and the environment.

"Well good luck," said me Mum. "So who would you vote for?"

"I won't vote. I want action."

"Don't we all? But you should still use your vote you know. Let the politicians do the acting." Me mum always voted Labour.

"But you've gotta keep going on at them cos once you stop shouting, they've won. They'll do nothing about climate-change, the sweatshops, the exploited. You've got to protest and fight."

"Paul, I agree with you. You just don't shout so loud when you're older."

"You're not old." He made me Mum blush.

Afterwards, he said:
"I like your mum. What does she do?"
"Saves troubled kids."
"Yeah?" He was impressed.

"Is he always like that?" she said.
"Like what?"
"You know - I like his passion but he's a bit, well, hyper."
He's mainly mouth, I said, and she said she'd had that feeling.

When I told McEwan I'd seen Karen for a fun night out, he said:
"Fuckinell, man. I thought she was with that Ian geezer.
"Yeah. So?" Bold boy.
I only saw her a couple more times that first term at college. One Friday night she came up Streatham Hill to meet me and McEwan in The Crown and Sceptre. She'd had a shit day, getting her Nokia nicked for the first time. I made her feel better by telling her about being jacked three times and McEwan made her laugh about the redistribution of wealth in London by street crime. He said he'd never been done over and never worried about it, so he never got done.
"Must be the way you look," said Karen.
"And what's that?" asked McEwan, touchy about his appearance.

"Well you look kind of grungey but unpredictable like you've got no money and don't give a shit but you just might kickbox em in the face or pull a gun."

He smiled, slid his hand inside his jeans and pulled out a two-finger pistol and shot her. I told her about McEwan pulling the water pistol on the old woman at the college registration.

"Poor woman," said Karen, giggling all the same. "You were lucky they didn't call the armed police."

"There was a shoot-out down the hill last week," I said. "In the newsagents. I saw the police taping it up. Man with gun walks into shop and blasts someone buying his fags and paper."

"Drug wars!" McEwan announces, fist up.

Time for another hard drink.

"So this is Streatham," she said, looking around the boring great bar room of The Crown and Sceptre, unimpressed.

"Well, a very small part of it," I said. "The real hotspots are up the road."

"Er, like what?"

"Like, like Ceasar's glittering nightclub." McEwan boasted, desperate.

"Ooh let's go!" she cried.

"Nah we're too young. Far too young."

"What do you mean?"

"Well, let's just say your old mate Ian would like it," McEwan said.

I laughed.

"Hey, he's not <u>that</u> old," she said, stabbing me hard.

"So where is the young man tonight?" McEwan nosed about.

"He's at home with his little family in North Wales," she said waving her arms about. "I'm just his London floozy. He chatted me up on a number 2 bus."

Bastard.

"The lurve bus!" McEwan in mega bass, making her giggle.

He and Karen were getting on fast. Too fast, cos basically I wanted her to like me, not him. I needn't have worried. McEwan had this thing about Brixton, didn't he?

"So what's it like living at the throbbing heart of south London, then?" he asked her, teasing.

"Brixton's brilliant," she said, falling for it. "Brilliant bars and clubs. And the Ritzy and the Academy. It's all there. Beats Bath, darling."

"So where's black Brixton in this brilliant fun palace? Nowamin?"

She pulled a very bored look.

"God, you still on about that? What about black Brixton? The kids are in the clubs, that's all I know. I don't know what you're getting at."

"It's da white colonisation of Brixton, dat's what. No jobs for blacks, innit. Police harassment. And da rich white kids crashing da bars and -"

"Oh come on, McEwan," she said, hands out, passionate. "Brixton's the strongest black culture in the UK. Even Lauryn Hill sings about Brixton and Kingston. It's that good. That's why Mandela came here."

"I was there," I reminded them. "I saw him."

"Da big bruvver." McEwan fist up. "Da Prince a Peace."

"And what _is_ all this with this fake rude-boy accent, McEwan?" Karen getting narked now.

"Dis talk all over London, Bath baby."

"Well I think it's just patronising. Trashy white boy stuff, if you ask me."

"But we's not asking you, is we? You know what I's saying?"

She stuck her tongue out at him then strongly advised him to stop going on about Brixton and things he didn't understand, and stick to his MacDonald's May Day riots and go and give Churchill a mohican or something.

"I did! That was me!" he shouted.

"Oh yeah."

"Yeah!" He meant it too. "I was there. It was _me_!"

He was pleading for our belief. We must have looked blank.

"You don't believe me, do you?"

"Course I do, mate," I told him, no problem. I liked believing his lies, especially the good ones, and lying back.

"_You_ don't though, do you?" he eyeballed Karen who wide-eyed him back,

smiling. Beautiful.

"Hey, let's go to Mass," she said, full of joy.

McEwan wasn't sure, after slagging off all the clubs in Brixton.

"Come on! You can't go on about Brixton and not live it," Karen said with a point.

"Yeah come on, mate," I joined in. "Let's go rolling, let's get hot."

He weighed it up. Some nights, McEwan decided the whole clubscene was a Ministry of Sound corporate compilation calamity, heartless and glossy, with the exception of NightSpot which had, of course, closed. Other nights, he just had to dance, didn't he, and when it came to it, he usually rolled with the rest of us, whatever the soul sacrifice. He pronounced:

"Course Mass ain't _real_ Brixton, is it? But hey who gives a fuck? Let's roll! Race ya! Race riot!"

And we ran and ran, all the way down Brixton Hill to Mass, gasping. The queue was mainly white and I could see McEwan preparing a big told-you-so speech, then a crowd of black boys swung in and shoved us up. Karen squeezed me, just for a moment, and I breathed her sweet shampoo.

Mass is music mayhem. McEwan was bored by most club music, all formula and no soul, but Karen and I liked the formula so who needs soul? He always wanted hip-hop and R&B, funky sounds with feeling, but we danced to anything that made you move and tonight we were all on drum and bass, on and on, like the DJ say: dance to give your body and soul for.

We were smiling and wet. Karen had to work three hours later. McEwan and I took her home and gave her big hugs and she said thankyou thankyou thankyou. So good. Oh yes.

STREATHAM COMMON 2001

McEwan's family had a party every New Year's Eve. He said you gotta come and meet the neighbours. I thought he was joking. Pleeease Alex, he said, very serious. Just for a while. We took some E's to make it swing.

In the pub he warned me about his family. His mother had a filthy temper and, being foreign, would kiss me and ask me personal questions, his young sister thought she was a celebrity model sadly and his father was basically a fascist. OK.

God it was cold. He lived the other end of Streatham up near the dark and windy common where the dogs howl and the houses have fancy front doors. We jumped high walls and deep holes and leapt through dangerous gardens to get to his house and charged in through the back door. In the kitchen his mother welcomed me warmly and made me feel wanted, rubbed my numb hands and made them glow. She wore black with crimson touches like flames and her ears sparkled in her big dark hair. Perhaps she was Irish. Or Spanish. Or possibly Indian. I asked him.
"What is your mother?"
"Complete mystery, mate."
"I mean - " Forget it.

I followed him, crowds of friendly neighbours cheering us on through the house. They shook my hand. McEwan got hugged and kissed. Then he swung a little girl round and started dancing to whatever the music was. His usual style of mad hands and feet, fast then slow, head down and trance-like, then up and all over the place. I watched him. Ate a fishy olive, nearly threw up and choked on the fizzy wine. Someone thumped my back and bits of olive and fish hit the carpet.

"Saved you," said the girl who hit me.

"Sorry. Those olives -"

"Are disgusting. I know. I've told me mum. She still gets them. She says people like them. Noone I know, I said. Older people, she said. Sick people maybe, yeah."

She talked very fast.

"You're Alex, aren't you? Paul told me about you. I'm Lizzie, his amazing sister. Wanna dance?"

"No thanks."

"Come on!" and she pulled me onto the floor.

I liked the red streak hair and the Kylie white dress.

"Didn't anyone tell you it was fancy dress?"

She knew what she was doing. She knew the disco party song, *Staying Alive, Staying Alive,* turned it into formation, clapping and spinning, and half the party joined in. Brave old ladies, drunk men and their children, arms in the air, legs out there. I was buzzing, creating. Then McEwan started heavy stomping, laughed at me across the circle and got me going. Helpless laughter. Dancing was impossible, walking was tough. I crawled over people with chicken legs and babies and spare ribs and walking sticks to get to the front door.

"Not in the porch, please. If you're going to be sick, go behind the bush," someone said, probably McEwan's dad, a bit sarci. I must have been holding my mouth to gag myself.
"The holly bush", he added.
"No thanks", I said.
I didn't need a chuck-up place. I wanted a big black sky and some stars. Space. Streatham Common. 2001. Massive.

Lizzie came out to save me.
"My dad thinks you're very drunk or epileptic."
"Uh."
"Are you?"
"No.....I'm....." I waved my hands around and creased up again.
"I see." She gave up.
When I stopped shaking, McEwan was there with my jacket and a bottle of champagne. Magic.
"Hey, bruvver, let's go and sparkle".

And we set off in search of fun in the community. Having no invitations or bribes and finding it hard to talk straight, we failed to persuade any doorman to welcome us into their pissy pub parties for some auld lang syne. Champagne on ice? Oh yes! But the ice rink was closed. The Go-Kart circuit was secure. What about the hospice up the hill? What a scream! So we leapt across the common wishing dog walkers and their dangerous dogs happy new years, slugging bubbles and chuckling merrily away. We were screaming out the party disco: *Ah ha ha ha, staying alive, staying alive.* We didn't know any more words. *Staying alive, staying alive.* Didn't need any more.

"The moon, man", he said, eyes fixed on it. From the top of the common you could see all the clouds moving thick and fast. The moon was so huge and the street lights so bright, the whole sky was silver and gold. Then the fireworks came swishing and banging across the commons from here to Wimbledon, Clapham and Tooting. We were flying. Higheeee.

McEwan sat in a tree and sang more snappy excerpts from *Staying Alive* to some passing girls who loved him for it. One of them danced a Flamenco number in return and we stamped and clapped and kissed and spread joy across the common.

Good night. Happy New Year. 2001! We love you. We love Streatham! Fuckinell.

BOYS DON'T TALK

"This is Matt, Alex," me Mum said. "He teaches on my course."
He turned up one night to take her to a movie and shook my hand.
"What course is that?" I asked.
"It's about working with families," he said. "Families who don't er work very well."
And they both laughed, nervous as hell.

Next day, she wanted to know what I thought of him.
"I dunno."
She told me they were seeing quite a lot of each other. Makes a change from Jane, she laughed. Jane was her old friend and companion. Poor Jane.

So me Mum started coming home late, clothes stinking of smoke, a bit pissed. Me own mum! I tried to feel deprived and neglected.
"Sorry I'm late, love. Did you eat?"
"Yeah. Two boxes of Sugar Puffs."
She used to want to know where I'd been and who with etc. But now she wasn't bothered, hardly noticed if I was out all night. I wanted to tell her that she could stay out too if she wanted, but I didn't.

Then Matt came for Sunday lunch and wanted to be matey while Mum did the finishing touches. He asked me about my A-levels and said he was crap at arty things but goes to movies to keep his imagination alive. As for French, he told me about Mum taking him to a French country dance club which he loved, having thought he couldn't dance at all, especially in French ha ha.

She cooked him roast lamb with white beans, even though she was usually vegetarian. She could eat lamb because they run around on hills.
"A classical Normandy dish," Mum explained.
"It's excellent, Pat," said Matt, impressed. "You're a very lucky bloke, Alex, to have a superchef mum."
"It's usually brown bread and chick peas," I said.
"Are you complaining?" she said. "No bread for you tomorrow."
She could be quite funny. Matt laughed loud. Then he went crazy about the chocolate mousse.

On their second bottle of wine they were talking deep, about how boys don't talk about personal things like feelings and fuck-ups. Mum said:
"I was talking to this new little boy at the unit, just trying to get to know him, and he put his finger on my lips and said in a loud whisper: DON'T EVER TELL ANYBODY ANYTHING. It was like his motto. Why not? I said. NOT TELLING YOU, he shouted at me and off he went, very pleased with himself."
Matt and I had a giggle at that, but Mum carried on her big theory.
"In my long experience of boys, they have to be really badly down before they'll talk, whether

they're hard cases or sad ones. Just like their dads of course. My father never talked about himself or his feelings except his prejudices. And Sean always had to get out of his head to talk sense. What about you two?"

Matt and I looked at each other. Maybe she had us sussed, us dumb boys. Then Matt spoke:

"Well I think us boys are a bit more open these days, don't you, Alex?"

"Yeah, sure," I said, whatever.

"When do you ever talk about your feelings then?" Mum said, not convinced.

"Well. Feelings are feelings. Not words." Being a smart arse.

"There you are you see," said me mum, proving her point to Matt. "Boys haven't changed. It's the old male stiff upper lip syndrome."

"The old stiff dick syndrome, more likely," said Matt.

And me mum clipped his ear.

"Can't take him anywhere."

"Well? Do you like him?" she asked me when he'd gone.

"He's OK," I said, and meant it. He was probably great for me Mum, clipping his ear and stuff. "Is he divorced?"

"Separated. He's got a family of his own."

"Thought so. He's got that look."

"Watch it, mate. So what about you then? Any more girlfriends?"

"No, I'm just sleeping around."

"Oh, that's OK then."

I hadn't seen Karen at all over the Christmas holidays, she was back in Bath. I badly wanted to see her. Trouble was she didn't always want to see me. I'd call her and she'd say "I'm seeing my friends tonight" like I wasn't one of them. I could hate her then, but I still wanted to be with her. Crap, isn't it? Then one time she had the nerve to say I should have a drink with her ageing lover Ian.

"He'd like to see McEwan and you again."

Bollocks.

THE KING OF SARDINIA

"<u>Course</u> boys talk," McEwan screamed at the top of Brixton Hill and jerked me up and down by my jacket. "Right, bruvver?"
I chewed my gum dumbly and he thumped me.

McEwan respected Ian, Karen's mature lover, ever since that night of love at first sight for little Alex, with Ian blagging about mountainside sex and playing dice to decide your life. So when he was staying at Karen's and she was working late one night, we three big boys went to the pub. Ian liked the King of Sardinia the other side of Brixton Hill cos it did Brazilian jazz and no rap crap, as he called all Brixton bar music. Moron.

He knew the barmaid, joked her about her new pink hair. He drank pints of Fosters and sneered at our bottles of Sol, in a fake thick scouser voice.
"Call them a man's drink? Them's for lassies, them are."
He leant forward and looked in your face, too close for comfort for me. But, let's face it, I already had a king-size aversion to Ian. He shagged Karen.

The barmaid was called Susie and she reminded him of his sad and distant youth, his first shag being a Susie, he said, on a country ramble in Wales. I didn't believe him. What he really wanted was <u>our</u> sex stories but no way were me and McEwan revealing our best hits, us being bashful boys and anyway sex is private, isn't it, <u>and</u> very rude and you don't wanna be talking rude with a forty year old wanker, do you? No. So instead we depicted for the old boy's pleasure some after-school group gropes and lesbian grungegirl parties, exaggerating a little. McEwan and me could blag nicely together and Ian was hooked. Was it a south London thing, he asked, this grungegirl sex business? Well, we said, sarf London is more common so everyone's more sexier ere, innit? Nice one, he said, chuckling, and then offered us some technical advice, man to boy.

"When you're with a girl, take it…slowly", he said confidentially. "Girls tease, right? They say yes, no, well maybe, but not now, later, they tantalise. So - when you've got them where you want them, keep them waiting, stretch it out till they're screaming for it. Alright? Slowly, remember. Works every time."

"Ya what?" I said, shocked and disgusted. "Me and McEwan only go fast-forward, mate. You get more in that way. Slow's a bit old romantic, isn't it? You see, Ian – " and I leant forward into his face "- sex has changed. Like food. Music. Broadband. Like fast fast fast."

McEwan was gawping at me. What was I gabbing about? Ian had a sick smile, not sure. I was laughing, wizzing. I charged on.

"What I mean, Ian, is – at our age, you gotta go fast, yeah? I suppose, when you're older, you gotta slow down. I can understand that. So you don't spill the beans or have a heart attack. When

I'm your age – yeah, maybe I go slow too, but now it's - " and I did some quick-fire karate chops with sharp sound effects.

McEwan screamed. Ian smiled and nodded knowingly.

"I was like that at your age."

You know what it's like when there's someone you hate and they keep saying things and you just have to argue with everything they say? You can't help it. And that's what happened with me and Ian. Basically, anything he said, I said the opposite. You know – he says it's been a really hot day and I say well I was bloody freezing.

So when we talked football and he said he supported Liverpool, I had to be Arsenal, didn't I? Palace wasn't flash enough. Trouble was, he always had an answer, didn't he, just like a teacher.

"Bloody frogs," he went.

Fucking racist.

After football, crisps. He rated McCoys, curry flavour.

"Can't stand them," I said, "Fat and wrinkly."

"Exactly," he said, proud. "Just like me."

Sick, eh? Then it was maths, his big subject.

"A perfect system of infinite yet logical calculation," he gloated.

"But maths only gives answers," I shouted brilliantly, "to questions no-one bloody well asks."

"But, Alex – does an answer always need a question?" he said, deep and slow, very pleased with himself.

Er. McEwan screamed at me being dumb. Bastard.

And then there was Brixton. Ian hated Brixton didn't he, so tonight I was Brixton's number one.

"The centre of the world," I said, "Where Africa, Europe and Asia unite."

"Unite and fight, you mean," he said. "It's bloody dangerous round here if you ask me, I never feel safe."

"But then you're not local are you?" I said, cutting.

"You mean asylum seekers aren't welcome here?" he said to shame me.

"So what oppressive regime are you escaping from?" McEwan asked him.

"My wife," he said to make us laugh but we didn't, so then he said, "Just joking, guys. Sorry, Jackie darling."

That was embarrassing. But then McEwan got all matey and personal and said to him:

"Did you know that little Alex here lusts after your lovely young Karen?"

"Piss off," I protested, but you could tell it was passion cos I was blushing.

I glared at McEwan. Coulda hit him.

"Don't worry, Alex, you're doing a grand job. Saves me entertaining her," said Ian. "You carry on dancing, mate. Hahaha".

Like I said, he always had an answer, didn't he? I went to the bog to spit.

McEwan was going on about global disaster and capitalist conspiracy, his usual crap, and I drifted off, dreaming of Karen, till Ian turned on me, just like a teacher putting you on the spot cos you're not paying attention:

"So what do _you_ think, Alex?"

And I just said:

"Well. Basically I think everyone should get a fair crack of the whip."

"But we're not talking about sex any more, Alex. Hahaha."

Now that wasn't very funny for a grown man, was it?

Then Karen arrives and I get edgy. Because Ian's here she's not really _my_ friend tonight, she's his. I hate that. They don't kiss or anything but Ian goes and gets a stool and sits close up to her. She looks knackered but nice, straight from work. She takes a gulp of his beer and smiles at McEwan and me. Those fucking eyes.

"How are you, Alex? Can I have a ciggie?"

She takes one of my fags. Ian doesn't smoke. At least I've got fags. She takes a deep drag. She's nervous, I'm nervous. McEwan kids her about her black and white hairy shoulder bag. He sniffs it, breathes it, stuffs it up his nose, testing.

"Moroccan goat," he announces.

"Well, Camden Market actually", she says.

"Ooo Camden Market actually is it?" he mocks in a posh voice and she sticks her tongue out at him then laughs like magic. Fuckinell.

"So where are we going? Telegraph, George IV, Mass?" I ask, provocative, wanting to see Ian's face curl but it doesn't cos Karen says:

"No thanks, no rave tonight, Alex, I gotta sleep."

Shit. Rejected for a pig. Ian looks very smug, like he's thinking: that'll show you, you little poser, you go and play with those rough Brixton kids while I go home and sleep with Karen and maybe have some very slow sex with her. That's what he's thinking, the bum. And just as I'm thinking how can I really hurt his smug red face, Karen's saying to me:

"But what about next week? Tuesday good?"

YES!

CLUBBING IN STREATHAM

"But there's no clubs in Streatham," she screamed.

"Remember Caesars?" I said. "They've got a brand new Ibiza Warm Up night."

"Mmm," she said.

"Then there's big boys lapdancing for women only on Wednesdays."

"Now you're talking. I'll take Celia."

"And - there's a deejay with a growing reputation Saturday nights at the Ice Rink. Known as The Iceman."

"I can't skate."

"Nor can I."

"So that would be foolish, wouldn't it?"

So scathing about Streatham she was. Just because she had the world-famous Mass and Fridge round the corner and music bars on every street, she'd started going on about how Brixton had all the nerve and culture and Streatham just had the High Road. What did she know? She'd just got out of Bath.

But she was right of course. Karen was a year older than me, big and brave, and I was her young dance-mate date for empty weekday nights. She took me to all the clubs and music bars around Brixton. She'd call and say: Mucky Duck? White Horse? Dogstar? Tonight. Then the flash spots in town she wanted to try, Herbal and Fabric, bigger and slicker. We zoomed in fast and got in cheap, lounged around on the pink leather sofas and black cubes watching the underwater movies to mad vinyl mixes. But Brixton was best, no question.

She got me to queue for hours for some weird techno girlband at the Astoria. Ladytron. Didn't rate them but I loved watching her dance. She showed me how. *I'm gonna be the one to step to you, put you in the mood to dance all night.*
"You dance heavy for a white girl," I shouted black-boy style and she loved it. And we sweated and breathed hot air and came home glowing on the night bus.

"She just uses you, mate," McEwan said.
"No problem, mate," I'd say. "Beats East Enders."
He was just jealous.

And she teased me. When I texted her once about sex, she texted me back:
"When you're seventeen, you aren't really serious." Just because she was eighteen, deadly serious and read French poetry.

She wasn't exactly my first crush. There was a girl in year 11 and we spent two weeks smoking and snogging on Clapham Common after the GCSEs. Then she vanished and I took the hint, no problem. But this feeling for Karen was more painful. And humiliating. First time I asked if I could stay the night, she said, "On the floor, mate." And when, as a joke but not really a joke, I said "Don't you do sex?" she said, "Look, just cos we go out together doesn't mean I'm gonna have sex with you. OK?"

"OK. OK," I said, reject boy.

"Yet," she added quietly, enticingly.

She said "yet". I'll never forget the look she gave me then. And the intravenous kick.

"So who's this Karen then?" me Mum asked.

"Just a girl."

"What else?"

"Lives in Brixton. Works in a bookshop -"

"Don't worry, love, I'm not jealous - yet."

Big word "yet". She laughed and thought about it.

"Actually, I could really get into the possessive mother role..." And she turned on me. "So who is this, this bookshop woman? Taking advantage of my young boy. Make up your mind, Alex. It's me or her."

"See you then, Mum."

"But Alex, my little Alex. How can you leave your poor mother, your own loving mother, for that...that runaround bookshop bitch."

And at that she slapped me violently round the head and I slumped across the sofa. Just playing. She could do a nice little drama, me Mum, when she wanted to. A frustrated soap star at heart. Big fan of Peggy Mitchell.

She suddenly says:

"Alex, I know you know about sex and all that, but if you ever need to talk, you know, about relationships, I do know a bit. I know boys find it hard to talk. But there's always Matt if you'd prefer to talk to a bloke. I know he'd be good."

I do a big nervous giggle. The idea of talking sex with the man who was shagging me Mum. I mean, really.

"Thanks Mum."

"The Brook Clinic in Brixton does free condoms."

"Mum."

"Sorry."

I didn't tell her that Karen didn't want sex with me. Yet. I didn't want to disappoint her. But sex with Karen was like clubbing in Streatham. It will take time.

COLLEGE DRAMA

It's a Mr Morrison masterclass on a scene from a Harold Pinter play. We're late in from smoking on the common. Mr Morrison waves at us to sit down in our usual back row seats and shut up. He's got people doing lines like -

"Do you like it?"
"What?"
"Your breakfast. Do you like it?"
"Oh yeah."
"I thought you would."
"Did you?"
"Yes. I knew it would be nice."
"That's nice."

McEwan says loudly, "This is kak."
Two girls go "ssshhhhh."
Morrison says, "Paul, you can share your insights at the end of the act. And mind your language."
The play restarts. McEwan looks at me.
"Mind your language," he whispers in a private Pinter piss-take.
"What?" I reply.
"I said mind your fucking language. That's what I said."
"I thought you did. That's not nice."
"What's not nice?"
"Your fucking language."
McEwan splutters too loud. Morrison comes up close.
"What's the problem, Paul?"

McEwan pulls his face of human suffering, gestures, pauses for dramatic effect and says:

"Sir - don't you get hacked off teaching us this white English Pinter crap?"

The rest of the class groan and mutter. Mr Morrison smiles and stands up straight and strong.

"Come on, Paul. Pinter's about power, domination, violence. I love Pinter. He's a Jew. He talks to me. You're not listening, man."

"But what about doing some black writers?"

"Paul, thanks for your concern, but first you read some black writers then you talk to me about black writers."

McEwan's stuck for a reply. The only black writers he knows are Rodney Smith and Puff Daddy.

"So Paul, if you want to stay, be quiet and listen," says Morrison, wise and sure. "But if you can't listen, then leave."

He leaves, doesn't he? In a rush, slamming the door. Unluckily he exits splat into the college Vice Principal, a woman dressed for business impressing a posse of inspectors. She asks where he's going with such urgency.

"The Windmill, Miss. Nice pub, near the pond. Excuse me," he says, and whooshes off to feed the ducks. He had no respect, that boy. None.

He called me later and said he'd written Mr Morrison an apology for his behaviour, telling him that he'd found Pinter so funny, he couldn't contain himself, in fact he was still laughing.

The next day, he received a letter from the Vice Principal who, following such rudeness, felt bound to act. She copied the letter to McEwan's parents who still had high hopes for their son. That was mean. Not that it made any difference, just made a family very stressed. He said his mum kicked his arse and his dad despaired.

Me, I'd had a giggle with McEwan at college but I could see it wasn't going to last. Just glad I wasn't him.

WISDOM IN CLAPHAM

Mr Morrison wanted to save McEwan from his A-level hell. He said, I'll buy you two a beer in The Calf, Clapham Village. Because he was a cool kind of guy. He wore pink shirts and black suits, gold earring and head close shaved. Our Head of English.

Sols all round then. Mr Morrison cared about us because we were rebels and radicals, he said, just like he'd been. He talked our language. He knew our stuff. But most of all he was vexed by McEwan's long struggle with the devils and of course his complete lack of achievement so far in the fantasy world of AS levels.

"What would help you to take it all more seriously, Paul?" He always called him Paul, unfortunately.
"God, that's a hard one, sir," McEwan said then got stuck.
"Look, I'm not trying to test you, man. You make your own decisions. But you can't carry on pissing about at college much longer. If you don't start delivering, it'll be on yer scooter, bruvver."
"On my scooter, eh?"
McEwan sucked hard on his fag and coughed lots. I couldn't tell if he was choking back hysteria or actually trying hard for Mr Morrison for whom, out of all the college staff, he had some respect. He tried to respond.
"Well. It's - I can't - I - "
Morrison interrupted his flow.

"Question authority, Paul – of course you should - but you still have a responsibility to yourself. Don't waste your talent just because you're angry with the adult world. I discovered you can influence things more by getting on and getting involved, not opting out all the time."

The wisdom gushed. McEwan stared at his half-empty Sol and said:

"I'm not interested in getting on right now. I'm too busy seeing to myself. Know what I mean, sir?"

Mr Morrison nodded seriously.

"I do, Paul. I was like you. I couldn't see the point. But as the night gets darker the stars get brighter. Remember that."

"Mmmm. Stars. Deep." McEwan said, sneaking a smile to me.

What?

When McEwan went to the bog to see the stars Mr Morrison said to me:

"You can help him, Alex. You seem to manage your own self-destruct impulses better than he does. And he has time for you. Trouble is, he's going to find himself up shit creek soon if he doesn't change his ways."

Trouble with Morrison was he preached at you, like he was always right, of course he was, like all fucking teachers, and you were wrong or just dumb. So I said, confidentially and respectful:

"I wouldn't go on about it too much, sir. He's got the message. I can tell. He likes to think things over in his own time. He's a very thoughtful boy."

He looked at me, not sure if I was taking the piss, then he said, " OK. I've said my piece, as my mother says."

On his second bottle, Morrison got personal and told us about being a Brixton rough boy and his new smooth life with his wife and kids and his big job as Head of English at the college.
"So where do you live now, sir?"
"Right here in leafy Clapham."
"Very nice, sir. Possibly a bit posh?"
He laughed.
"Brixton's too fast for me now, man. Much too fast. I need space to think my green thoughts in the shade."
"Come and chill in Streatham," I said.
"I do! I take my kids to the ice rink and watch them skate."
"Not for you, sir?"
"Like I say, bruvvers - ice is great if you skate, shit if you slip".
"Very wise, Mr M."
"And when I read the South London Press about the latest shootings, I thank God for our home in sunny Clapham and I pray for Coldharbour Lane."
"You gotta watch out, sir."
"Don't worry, man. I've got a bullet-proof soul."
He had a big laugh.

"So did you do the Brixton riots, sir?"
McEwan was excited by the legendary local history of urban terror. Mr Morrison was amused.
"I didn't start them, man!"

"Bet it was good though." McEwan wide-eyed.

"It was scary, man. I was only 14. But I had to be there. I was angry, like all the kids. Angry at the cops. Angry at the world. And angry with our parents, their generation, you know? This was the 1980's, remember. It was us young blacks standing up for ourselves and fighting. We hadn't done that before."

"Respect!" shouted McEwan, fist up.

"That's what we wanted. Not middle-class whites raving at Rock Against Racism concerts."

"My Mum saw The Clash in Brockwell Park," I said.

"Great. But they weren't black. We had to do it for ourselves. Brixton was angry. Twenty years after the riots, it's got respect and it's moving fast."

"And going <u>white</u> fast, too," said McEwan, pointing the finger. "White kids from Bath and places moving in, taking over."

I got the dig, flicked a V at him. Mr M said:

"Brixton won't ever go white. It's not like Notting Hill. Brixton's a real community. Black and white and united. Allright?"

He laughed his big laugh and touched fists all round.

"But if Brixton's so great, why do you leave it, sir?" McEwan really wanted to know.

Mr M got serious and loud.

"I'll tell you why not. Because I'm a parent and Brixton is tough. I don't want my children growing up where men are blasting each other over drug deals, black boys are leaving school with nothing and girls are three times more likely to get pregnant under age. Brixton's still got big problems. I'll teach their kids every day, I'll do my bit, but I don't have to <u>live</u> it, you know? You make your own decisions what's best for you and your young ones. Black or white. Right?"

McEwan was looking perplexed. Morrison was emotional. McEwan had got it wrong. He said:

"I didn't mean - " and got stuck.

Morrison helped out, leaned back, lightened up, stopped the preaching.

"Hey look, boys, we shouldn't be vexing ourselves over Brixton. You two should be grooving back home in Streatham. Enjoying yourselves."

"But when you think about it, sir," I said, keeping it bright, "Streatham without Brixton is like - "

"A fag without a light," said McEwan still holding an unlit ciggie.

"Yeah, like - hip and no hop."

"Drum and no base."

"And Paul without Alex?" Mr M wondered.

"Yes! In other words, sir, a complete bag of shite!"

Morrison was chuckling, but puzzled.

"You're a funny pair, you two. And I've got to go home. To my cosy Clapham nest."

He got up, shook our hands.

"Remember, all I'm saying is - use your talents. And use your teachers. Including me. Do that and you'll both be stars. Big stars. Right?"

"Thanks, sir."

"And thanks for the Sol, sir. Love to the family," I said.

"Yeah. They don't listen to me either."

"Slap 'em, sir."

McEwan went quiet, then angry. He didn't like it. Morrison had shown him up, like he didn't know what he was talking about when it came to real life and being black and Brixton going white and shit. They were McEwan's delusions, that's all, like his fantasies. He wanted to be da cool white rude boy. But to be real Brixton, real rude boy, real cool, you had to be black, and he wasn't, was he? What a fuck-up. Sad really.

At least he didn't go on about Brixton after that. Didn't go there much either. But I did.

KISSING KAREN

I could see her outside Brixton tube, waiting for me with the preachers, the dealers, the hawkers and the beggars. She hadn't seen me. She looked great, jeans, tight white top. I came up behind her and kissed her neck and she back-heeled me fucking hard with her steel heel on my shin. I nearly crumpled.
"Don't do that, you creep. You just don't do that", she said, tense as shit.
I wanted to scream fuck you in her face but didn't. People were staring and smiling. So I smiled too, like it was fun not pain.

We started walking, me limping, hurt and silent.
She said, "Look, I just don't like being kissed by someone who comes up behind me in the middle of Brixton. Can you get that?"
"I get it."
"And I <u>hate</u> having my neck kissed."
"OK."

Somehow we went and danced. Down a deep techno ghetto, she called it. Some place in town I didn't even notice. I killed the pain in my leg with strong lager and pills. Eventually she asked me how my damaged leg was and hugged me hard.
"You donkey bitch," I said. "You nearly broke it."
"Merde." She often swore in French and Greek cos it sounds exotic and her granma won't understand.

She lifted my leg up and stroked it and kissed the lump. It fucking hurt.

But I liked her. Really liked her. I was getting used to seeing her and thinking about her when I wasn't with her. I don't think she thought about me much. I was just someone to go dancing with and get home with when she had noone else to go with. She'd get cold waiting for the night buses and we'd hug and shake each other and jump up and down to get warm. She appreciated that.

Tonight on the 159, she told me how she met Ian. I didn't want to know, thanks, but she told me. She was sitting on top of a number 2 and picked up a Big Issue thinking someone had left it but the man on the next seat - Ian - said yes of course you can read it and she said sorry I thought someone had left it but he insisted she have it anyway and they laughed and got talking about their shared passion for homeless people and he said let's meet again and start an affair and they did. He told her later that it wasn't his Big Issue at all. The bum.

I kept picturing this little upstairs scene and his patronising chat-up lines as he leaned across the front seat of the fucking number 2. "We're so lucky to have homes to go to," he'd say, like a saint. "I just thank God my university wants me to go on teaching or I'd be on the streets selling the Big Issue myself." And she fell for it. Fucking fell for it.

I didn't understand her taste in men and boys.

"I know you don't like me being with Ian. I just like him, that's all."

"I never said anything about him."

"Exactly," she said. And she kissed me. "He can't dance like you, you know."

But she still had sex with him. That hurt. Like my leg.

"He's old enough to be your dad." I had to say it one day.

"No," she said, hurt and annoyed.

"How old is he then?"

"Thirty-four."

"He looks about fifty."

"Oh shut-up, Alex. That's pathetic. I like him, OK? And I like you. I really want us to be friends. And if you don't like Ian, I'm sorry. That's how it is."

Karen was straight-talking, her hand slicing the air. Tension on the hectic upper deck, nothing more to say, looking opposite ways. Then she tried to lighten up and stroked my leg.

"I didn't know you cared so much," she said.

I still couldn't look at her, but when the bus swung into Brixton Hill I swallowed my pride and took a chance she might take pity on me. I said:

"Can I come back with you?"

"Sorry Alex." A pained look. "Ian's there. I'll call you."

She kissed me quickly and rushed downstairs.

Fuck.

OK, OK, so I was young and foolish and proud. Like she and I were just doing kids' stuff, going dancing and kicking the shit out of each other, and then she goes home to be cool and adult with her <u>real</u> lover aged 34. I had to make her take me more seriously, make her just want <u>me</u>. But she was <u>so</u> mature and complicated, wasn't she? She saw me in Clapham once with a girl from college and I hoped she'd be badly jealous but she just said, "Who was the girl? She looked really sweet." Like I was her kid brother. Bitch.

TROUBLED KIDS' PARTY

I was in a bad mood for days after that night of pain. I didn't call her and she didn't call me. She had more important things to do than piss about with a boy with a sore leg, didn't she? It had come up in a massive bruise, heart-shaped and blue. I stared at it and poked it and felt the pain. Mum caught me with my jeans pulled up, leg out, bruise shining.

"How did you get that?"

"Karen kicked me when we were dancing. An accident. It's nothing."

"That Karen's just a bleedin clumsy gel." Mum in her Peggy Mitchell mode again. "No manners, no respect, those young gels. And they can't dance, just ain't got the steps - "

She could have gone on then she saw I wasn't laughing. She turned into a nurse and went and got the arnica, the right stuff for bruises, and rubbed it in. Ouch. She knew I was hurting, didn't ask any more.

Her troubled kids unit was having a party and she asked me and McEwan to go and add some sparkle to the occasion.

"Just for an hour or two. The kids will love to see you. They're always asking about you."

"Yeah?"

She worked, you'll remember, in an adolescent unit, comforting the troubled kids.

"There's no drinking, of course," she said.

"Sex and drugs?"

"Don't you dare."

I told McEwan.
"So what's up with these kids?" he asked.
"So stressed they get ill," I said.
"No problem," he said, like he was going to put an end to their troubles for good and all.
"There's no drink or drugs or sex," I said.
"Poor kids. Let's give them a night to remember."

Me Mum got a bit nervous about it, worrying what to wear so she didn't look like she cared. She said her young man Matt would be there.
"Say hello to him, won't you, love?"
"Course I will. Hello Matt. Easy."
"I want everyone to have a good time. No traumas, no trouble."
"Yeah, yeah. It'll be fine. McEwan and I are there, remember."
"Yes," she sighed.

McEwan was high and lively that night. He wanted to meet the sad kids and show them he cared. He dressed up for them. Big purple shiny shirt, particularly sharp hair. After a couple of spliffs and some shots of vodka from a Lucozade bottle, he was smiling all over. Me, I felt edgy, paranoid, not right. Didn't want to go in.
"Don't you dare do any smoke or vodka in there," I said.
"Alex. I know what to do. I'm a troubled kid myself, remember."
I didn't trust him.

The music was loud rap and the dance floor was empty. A few groups sat round the edges, under the tied-up balloons, staring at us. I wanted me Mum. A girl shouted out, louder than the music:

"Alex! Alex! Come here." She knew my name. She was with me Mum. We went over, McEwan stopping to do a few shuffles and spins in the middle of the floor. Me mum introduced us. A man with a beard and boots like he'd just climbed a mountain: Brian the boss nurse. A skinny young woman, Sarah, with long red hair and a black vest with a shiny tree on it. And on top of her, much bigger than her, the girl who shouted, with heavy duty make-up and slicked hair, smoking in and out very fast. She couldn't stop. A troubled girl.

"This is Aisha," said me mum. "Aisha, this is Alex and Paul."

Aisha screamed and buried her face in Sarah's tight tits.

"Hey, Aisha," said Sarah, "You said you wanted to meet Pat's son and his friend. Don't go all shy on us,".

"Piss off, Sarah,"

"Language, Aisha," said me Mum.

"Arseholes, Pat," shouted Aisha.

"Cool it, Aisha." A quiet warning from the boss man.

"Don't worry, Aisha," said McEwan boldly. "I wanna cuss and scream all the time too."

"Do ya?"

"Yeah. I go wwwaaaaaahhh!" and he leapt high and punched the sky with both fists.

Aisha screamed and laughed at him, curling up to Sarah.

"He's mental, him. He's mental."

"Come and have some food, Paul," me Mum said, worried what he might do next, and guided me and McEwan to safety in another room. "Don't be put off by Aisha. She's just very excited."

"Yeah, so am I," said McEwan, goggle-eyed, sticking his finger in the humus.

Me Mum laughed nervously.

"Thanks very much for coming, by the way, Paul. I really appreciate it."

"My pleasure entirely, Mrs Alex. And my duty. I wanna do my bit."

"Do call me Pat, Paul," she said, but he never did.

At the buffet table we met a boy with a round yellow face like the moon with spots and a school blazer, buttoned tight.

"Hello. I'm Anthony." He spoke slowly and moved carefully.

"Hi, Anthony. How are you?"

"Not very well actually."

"Oh dear. What's up, mate?" McEwan was concerned.

"My mother says I've got an old head on young shoulders. I worry too much."

Before McEwan could start slagging off Anthony's mother, I got in the way and said:

"Hello. I'm Alex. Pat's son."

"Pat? She's nice, Pat. She's very nice. I like Pat."

Strange hearing him talk about me mum like that. In fact, he wouldn't stop.

"Pat's your mum is she? You're very lucky, Alex."

"Yeah."

"I wish Pat was _my_ mum. She's so nice. She talks to me - "

"Mmmm, I love celery so much I could eat it all," shouted McEwan, shoving a whole stick down his throat and choking, to shut old Anthony up.

"I don't eat vegetables. I just like crisps and ham," said Anthony, while McEwan choked. "And I'm not supposed to eat ham."

McEwan was turning hysterical, laughing and gasping dangerously. I badly needed to escape this strange boy who loved my Mum and ham. I slapped McEwan hard on the back and stuck my fist in his kidneys. He spluttered and choked up.

"No more celery for you, mate. Excuse us, Anthony. My friend needs help."

"Goodbye Alex. You're very lucky, you know. I love Pat. I wish – "

"Yeah I _know_." A bit snappy, I couldn't help it. "But she's _my_ mum, allright?"

I led McEwan back to the dance floor, feeling bad and stressed. He was creased up, trying to speak.

"More food, Alex," he gasped. "I need food."

"No you don't. That boy's in there."

He creased up again, in a ball on the floor.

A boy, small and white, and a girl, small and brown, came up to us, holding hands. They were like miniature adults, tough and deeply troubled.

"Got any spare fags?"

McEwan gave them a couple.

"Don't inhale though," he said. They didn't laugh. The girl said:

"See that boy over there in the red MacKenzie shirt?" We all stared at a boy standing on his own by the wall. "He killed another boy, He's only 13. He don't talk to noone. He scares the shit outa me."

McEwan and I gawped.

"Got any puff?" her little boyfriend said to the floor.

"Puff? What's that? Puff. Don't know about that," said McEwan.

"No, definitely not. No puff," I said, very definite.

The girl had cuts up her hands and wrists. The boy had "BB" written on his neck in biro. McEwan asked what it meant.

"It's my mark," he said.

"Bum Boy," the girl giggled.

"Fuck off," said the boy.

"So what is it then? Big Bollocks? Big Bang?" says McEwan and shoots him.

"It's his initials," says the girl, giggling some more. "Bobby Bond."

"OK. Well then, Mr Bond, Mr Bobby Bond, where is the boys' bathroom, please?" asks McEwan, American movie star.

And the little lovers led him away. I didn't trust him.

Someone must have had a quiet word with the DJ from Peckham who was a very cool uncle of one of the kids and only did rap. Please don't be hip, be shit, think of the nurses, do Abba for God's sake. So he did. Two kind women got up, waving their arms about trying to get some of the kids up and active, with no success. When they reached out to McEwan as he strolled back on his own from the bog, he couldn't resist their plea. The women beamed, kids stared, and Abba sang. This was his big dance. He stretched up to heaven and down into hell. He got the spirit of Abba completely. The room swung into action, kids jumped up, copying him, laughing and stomping. *Mama Mia, here I go again.* The DJ lined up another old dancefloor classic. Madonna. McEwan jerked and rolled and didn't stop smiling. *Hey Mr Deejay put a record on, I wanna dance with my baby.* Everyone wanted to dance with McEwan. The party had connected.

"Allo Alex," me Mum's young man Matt the psychologist shook my hand. "Quite a raver, your friend. Not in the mood yourself?"
"Not tonight thanks, Matt."
"I'm more of a soul man myself," he said. "Mary J, Macy Gray…er…Marvin Gaye."
He wanted to impress.
"Sure," I said. "And what about that French country dancing you told me about?"
A sad activity for a soul man, and he blushed.
"Yeah, but your mum's more into that than I am really. I just give her something to hold onto," he blagged. "Ever seen it ? The woman swings around the man, round and round. I keep her from spinning off into space. First time I did it I got so dizzy watching her go round, I fell over."
"Yeah?"

We watched McEwan go crazy to Britney Spears with twenty troubled kids.

"So what do you think of this place then?" asks Matt.

"Thank God I don't live here."

"Your friend seems quite at home."

"He's fairly disturbed."

When James Brown screamed, McEwan screamed, and everyone screamed. After some mad formation footwork with his troupe of troubled kids, he started a shaky conga snake round the room, shaking arms up here and legs out there, and everyone followed. Even me Mum was in there, beating it, shouting at us. Matt had no choice, being a soul man. Come on Alex, he said, shoving me into the line. *I feel good, dadadadadadada, I knew that I would, dadadadadadada.*

When the snake rattled and rolled out into the garden, they found little Bobby Bond looking after his girl who had flaked out in a flower bed. Me Mum was kneeling by her. The dancing had stopped, a crowd had formed, but James Brown kept on screaming from inside. *I feel good dadadadadadada.*

"What's she taken, Bobby?" someone was asking him in the face.

"Nothing. She just fainted. Honest." Bobby lied.

A hand pulled me away.

"I need a drink," McEwan gasped in my ear.

I said goodbye to Matt and we left.

I knew exactly what had happened.

”Did you give those kids a smoke, McEwan?”

“Yeah, yeah. They needed a lift. Did you see her hands? She was desperate.”

“You are fucking crazy. You’re fucking about with a young kid who’s ill. I told you no drugs.”

“She’ll be fine, had a bit too much vodka that’s all. Don’t worry, mate, it’s really good draw.”

I hit him hard. Then I laughed alot.

RESPONSIBILITY

The day after the troubled kids' party, me Mum woke me up and made me sit down and have breakfast with her. She was staring out the window waiting for the toast, no chit-chat and no radio. Not a good sign. I asked her how the girl who collapsed was. I wanted to know she hadn't died.

"She's alright. She and Bobby had taken some cannabis. And alcohol. She just blacked out."

There was more to come, I could tell. She knew the full story.

"Bobby told us that your mate McEwan gave them vodka and a spliff. Did you know that?"

"He told me afterwards. I'm sorry, Mum. I told him he'd been really dumb. He thought he was doing them a favour."

"Bloody hell, Alex. Is he that stupid?" She shouted, looked me straight in the eyes. "I am so angry with him. He seemed such a great guy, dancing with everyone, getting the whole thing going. They loved him. Then he does this. Doesn't he understand how vulnerable these kids are? They're only twelve, for God's sake. Doesn't he know it's wrong?"

What could I say? Didn't know the answer anyway. I ate my Coco Pops. She said:

"I'm going to talk to his parents."

"No, don't. He's in enough trouble with them already. They're teachers or something. They'd kill him."

"They're going to find out soon enough, you know."

"How?"

"Brian the manager may have to involve the police. We can't just ignore it, Alex."

"One spliff?"

"Look, I know we all use the stuff, but it's still actually illegal and he was supplying children, for God's sake. Kids who need protecting. I told you no drink or anything, didn't I? I thought I could trust you to be responsible."

Responsibility made me sick. She shoulda known that. But she was steaming, no question, staring out the window and breathing hard. I wanted to escape.

"Is he always that manic, your Paul McEwan? Does he ever get really down?"

"I dunno."

"I bet he does. Watch him. He might need help himself."

She wanted to talk to the bad boy about what he'd done. But she never got the chance. He never came round after that. Shamed.

I blamed her and she blamed me. It was like McEwan had committed some crime against humanity and I hadn't stopped him. Kids smoke and drink, don't they? Anyway, I didn't tell McEwan about me Mum's reaction at first, thinking she'd made her point and that was that, water under the bridge, tomorrows another day, give the boy a chance. Then, a couple of days later, she told me that her boss Brian, the man in the mountain gear, had asked McEwan to meet him, just to talk, before he decided whether to inform the police. Unfortunately McEwan couldn't be arsed to turn up for this meeting, so the police were now on the case: to teach McEwan a lesson.

I called the mad boy to warn him.

"What's the horror story? It's legal in Lambeth now isn't it?" He'd heard the news.
"You get a caution for possession, that's all," I said. "But supplying children is something else. You could hang, mate."
He choked then came alive again.
"Let the bastards come," he shouted. "I'm clean. You can have all my drugs tonight."
"No thanks."
"You're a real mate."
"Not me, mate."
"Well fuck you then."
"Good luck, McEwan."

I was not well pleased with me Mum. I was sick of her trouble and grief. First Karen, and now me mum. When I came in one evening and hardly noticed her, she said:
"I know you're angry with me, Alex, but we can still talk, can't we?"
"Mmm."
"I know you don't like it, Alex, but if Paul can't take responsibility for what he did, harming young kids with drink and drugs, there are consequences he

has to face. The police will probably give him a warning."

I was sick of her being right and I was sick of troubled kids. And women. Especially my caring, responsible Mum. What about me? Yeah? So I shouted at her:

"You invited us, Mum. It was a party, right? And we're boys, right? BOYS. Not bloody adults. And not bloody nurses. And I HATE your bloody troubled kids, OK?"

Slammed my bedroom door. Turned the music up fucking loud. My dad's music. Clash or XTC or something. Mad and bad and angry. I wanted him. I wanted me Dad.

DAD DREAM

Saturday in March, my dad's birthday. He would have been forty. Mum'd been to Sainsbury's for some warm doughnuts and woke me up for a birthday breakfast. I stuck a candle in a doughnut and we let it burn.

She told me a dream she'd had about him. He'd come alive again specially for his big birthday and brought lots of presents to show Mum but she wasn't interested in the presents, she just wanted him to stay and cuddle and talk but he wouldn't stay still, wriggling and slipping, she couldn't hold him, and he disappeared, smiling and winking at her. But he'd left all the presents, so she yanked one open and a joke snake sprang out at her. She woke up screaming, then crying, then laughing.
"I wanted <u>him</u>, not his bloody presents." And she hammered the table so the candle fell off the doughnut and went out.
"Did you tell him about Matt?" I said.
"No, he'd be jealous. Dead jealous."

She used to talk about him a lot when I was younger because she wanted me to know things about him, but not so much lately. I didn't tell her I'd been thinking about him alot. She said:
"Do you ever wonder what it would have been like to have a dad around?"
"Weird weekends doing Palace and PC World?"
"Football maybe. Computers no. He was a punk rebel remember not a techie. He couldn't mend his

own push bike. He'd have made you laugh though. Snakes on springs every day with him."
"Did he pogo?"
"Yeah. So did I, till I got too big with you. But Sean carried on partying. He'd been at The Marquee the night he died. He ended up at someone's flat in Kings Cross. Fourth floor of one of those old estates with bricked-up balconies, and he couldn't resist walking the wall. He was wrecked, silly boy. Silly, silly boy." She choked a bit, then she laughed. "I'm still angry with him."
"Why?"
"Because he left me. And you. And because he couldn't accept responsibility. But that's how he was. You know, he really wanted me to have the baby - you - but it didn't change him."
"Did he want to die?"
"No. The opposite. He couldn't grow up. He was twenty-three, with a six-month old baby, and he was still pissing about as an ageing punk. He was really chuffed with you, though. He insisted we call you Alex because he thought you looked like Malcolm MacDowell doing Alex in Clockwork Orange. But I told my mum we named you after Alexander the Great and she said ooooh really? he'll be a handful."
I saw Clockwork Orange when it was reissued but I didn't rate it much. Mum was disappointed, cos it had shocked her. But then, she couldn't watch Trainspotting after the dead baby.

I dreamt about my dad soon after Mum's dream. We were at a party and being crazy together - he was my age but still my dad - just me and him, like mates. He was in mad punk kit with a scarf round his head like a gypsy, leaping about and balancing on balconies. I tried to warn him but I couldn't speak.... I woke up, stressed. I didn't tell Mum.

I wanted him to stay around. I could have asked him what to do about Karen and her old lover and how to move him on. He's the main thing I can get soft about, my dad. I've got his old records. Clash, Pistols, Ramones, Generation X, Jam, Bowie, Costello, Velvet Underground. When I play them I try to think what he'd be thinking when <u>he</u> played them. I know it's weird but I feel like I know him and I know I'd like him. You know?

And I know he'd like McEwan. Another wild boy in a big mess.

McEWAN IN BIG MAC MESS

McEwan was my mate, sure, and I wanted to see him right, but it was getting hard. One day he was up and flying, the next he was down and deep. And tonight he was grounded after a visit from the Streatham drug squad - a nice man who McEwan was convinced used to be in The Bill and who told him to report to the cop shop next week to get charged or cautioned. His mother was demanding a public flogging, his father couldn't talk.

He escaped and legged it to the pub. Poor boy was in a right mess. Crumpled old T-shirt, hair screwed up, big silly smile.
"Alex! The cops were brilliant. He asked me where I got my stuff from and I said you."
"Oh yeah?"
"Yeah. And he wanted to know what drugs I liked best so I said I'm strictly organic, me, well within Lambeth rules, oh yes, none of these modern chemical products for me. Oh no."
"Course not."
"Then he asked me why I'd given the little kids a spliff and I said to cheer them up and he said he knew these kids were sad cases but I should know better and set an example and I said yeah I know but I'd heard it was OK in Lambeth now and I'd got confused. So he explained that supplying drugs to children is just not on and I should have known that and he thought I'd get a caution so I was on police records and if I ever came to their notice again, they'd throw the book at me."

"Ouch."

"Didn't even search my room. I'd hidden the stuff in my dad's tub of Brylcream so the dogs couldn't sniff it."

"They had dogs?"

"No, just our cat. And she was totally out of it."

On his second pint of Stella, his mobile rang. He said:

"Course I'm OK... I just need some space, Dad...Trust me... I've gotta think things through...I know you do...Thanks."

He ended the call, leaned right back and stared at the ceiling, closed his eyes.

"You allright, mate?" I said.

"No I'm fucking not."

"Parents?"

"Sick. Me dad's in tears. Me mum's drunk and threatening to smash me up. Lizzie's screaming at them."

"Families eh?"

"Fuck you up good and proper, mate." He waved his arms about to get free, then he leaned across and said, quiet and confidentially: "What happened to <u>your</u> dad, Alex?"

He hadn't asked me that before. Noone did really.

"Well. He fell off a balcony doing a mad balancing act. Died a drunk punk."

McEwan was excited.

"Did he? What a way to go, man! Whaaa – " Then he got embarrassed, remembered it was my dad, and went all serious. "Sorry, mate. Bad time. Bad time."

"I never knew him."

Pause for deep thought in the mega-bass soul of the bar's sound system.
"My parents say I'm a danger to myself." One of his laser looks. "What do you think?"
"Yeah. Major disaster. Total eclipse."
"Fuck off."

He stubbed out his fag and stared at it.
"What's your mum think about me now? Now that I've done bad with her sad kids."
"Look, can't we talk about global warming?" I was tired of his troubles.
"No. What does she think?" Face in mine. "I like her. I wanna know."
He was getting pissed and insistent. God knows what else he was on already.
"OK. She thinks you were stupid and irresponsible."
"I hope she appreciates -" banging his glass down on the table – "that we went to that fucking party out of charity…to do good…not to corrupt her sad kids but…but to give them a nice time. I danced with them. I made them happy. Didn't I? And now I'm under fucking investigation."
"Don't blame me Mum for that. She's concerned about you."
"I bet she is. Everyone is. Except you."
What did he want? Sympathy?

He slumped, deep in shit. He started drinking Smirnoff Ice. He was slipping around and slurring.

93

I needed help, a break. Me Mum's hero, Beckham, flashed on the big screen.

"Hey, man. The greatest living Englishman," I said to lighten up.

"What?"

"Beckham. Sir David. Bending it."

He didn't even look. Beckham scored.

"Wanka," he mumbled.

"Me Mum's hero."

"She would, wouldn't she? And you agree with her, don't you? You always agree with your women. Especially that Karen."

"I fucking don't."

"And – she's not pretty. That Kaz."

"What? What's pretty got to do with it? You're just jealous cos you ain't got a girl."

"They can't keep up with me, mate. I'm too - "

Yeah, there was no word to describe him, his hand waving about above his floppy head. I wanted to kick him. He said:

"She likes it all ways doesn't she, that Kaz? Young and old. Man and boy. Ian and Alex."

"Shut-up, will ya?"

"Seriously mate…how can you share her with that Ian?"

"I'm not going to."

"You dumping her?"

"No. But I'm gonna make him shift his fat face."

"Yeah?" He was intrigued.

"Yeah. You gonna help me?"

"Not me, mate. Never mess with people's love affairs. You gotta sort it. I just do the big boys - MacDonalds and Microsoft and – " he waved his arms about in search of more enemies and knocked his bottle over instead.

I had to get him out.

"Hey, let's go somewhere."

"But we're here, aren't we? What do you mean, dickhead? Go where?"

"I dunno. Mass. Hobgoblin. Dogstar. Do you good. Go rolling. Shake it up, boogie down, sweat it off."

"Sometimes, Alex, you can be so fucking... dumb, man. Here's me in deep shit and all you can think of is, is…raving." He leans across the table, elbows in beer, soft and sincere. "I'm in a mess, Alex. Not just a bitpisstoff. My parents are cracking up, the police are on my case, the college want me out. And you say lezdance!"

"So you just sit in the fucking – what the fuck's this pub called? - and get completely dumb-arsed juiced, do ya?"

"Well that's what you do when you're fucking fucked up, isn't it? Not fucking DANCE."

We both stop, look and laugh. He grabs my hand. Bruvvers.

"Look, mate, I'm too mashed to go anywhere. I just wanna talk. Off the chest, know what I mean? See these? "

He pulls up his sleeves and shows me his arms. Cuts, criss-cross, star-shape cuts, and burns, ciggie burns. One of them is wet and gooey and blistered.

"What the fuck do you do that for?" I feel sick.

"It's just skin graf, man." Mad smile, flashing it in my face.

"How long you been doing that?"

"Not long. But don't tell anyone, will ya? You're my mate, Alex. Wanna see my legs?"

"Piss off."

I shove him away, disgusted.

I go quiet, can't help it, can't think, can't look at him. He suddenly decides he wants to go and see Karen's Ian for whom he has a lot of respect. That's OK with me cos I need help too, so I call Karen to see if fat Ian's there to give the boy some ancient wisdom. No Ian, but there's always Karen. I tell her McEwan's in a mess and can I bring him round anyway cos he can't go home like this and she says OK if he's homeless and harmless.

"He just needs a floor."

"One night only?"

"One night only."

"And you clear up the sick."

God she was hard.

He insists on getting a MacDonalds, cos he feels so disgusting. I can't believe it, he must be bad. He hasn't eaten in days, he says, and hasn't had a MacDonalds since he was 12. He drops most of it down his shirt. I push him onto a bus and he tells me and the other passengers on the downstairs deck:

"I can't stay at home any more, Alex. My parents jus don't understand. It's, it's time to join the circus, bruvver. Time to, to roam."

"Where, mate?"

"Wherever the sunshine takes me, bruvver. Wanna come?"

A Jamaican gran nearby chuckles and says, "I'll come wid you, darlin!"

And he kisses her, sweet and sloppy.

When Karen opens the door, he yells "Kaz! Kaz baby!" and hugs her. She goes, "Ugh, what's all that down you?" and he says, "Big Mac, darling. Disgusting ain't it?"

She pushes him away, well disgusted.

"But Kaz, Kaz, KAZ. Listen. Come here. " He flings an arm round her and holds her close. "Lizzen. Don't let this boy here…Alex…leave ya. He's…he's too good to lose and… he's almost your own age… Alright?"

He nods and winks at me like he's sorted it with Karen for me.

"Alright," she says and gives me a brilliant naughty smile.

"Alright then." He let's her go then sways into the bog and crashes out in the bath with a towel. What a mess.

When I tell her about the kids and the spliff and the police, she just laughs.

"He's mad, that boy. Tutto matto."

"Yeah. But he'll be alright," I say, not believing it.

I didn't tell her about his cuts and burns. It was too sick, too personal. I wanted to forget it. I was thinking about me and Karen now, not him. I'd had enough of him. I wanted the attention now, <u>me</u>,

Alex. And it was so good to be with her, on her own in her flat. She made me a coffee, asked how my leg was. I showed her the heart-shape bruise and she stroked it, really sorry about that kick. She actually let me sleep with her that night, not much else, but getting closer eh?

I wake up thinking about the gooey cuts up McEwan's arms. When does he do it? What does he use? I don't want to know. I just want to tell Karen, someone, but I can't, cos I'm his mate.

BRIGHTON

It was Easter holidays and sometimes Streatham can piss you off. I called Karen and she said it's my day off tomorrow and I said yes! let's quit the city and go to the sea and she said yes! I've always wanted to go to Brighton. Yes! Then McEwan called and said what are you doing tomorrow? And when I told him he said could he come too? I said: no! But he still came.

He badly needed friends and sanity, he said, have mercy. His parents were deconstructing him, demanding total transformation. I gave in. Karen said, "He better behave himself."

The poor boy insisted on buying us vanilla steamers on Clapham Junction to have with the big bag of little sponge cakes he'd brought as a treat. He gobbled about ten then stood up and had a major spasm to shake the crumbs off his shiny suit. Karen watched him and said:
"Strange choice of clothes for the seaside, McEwan."
"Do you mind? This is my Brian Jones suit," McEwan announced, serious.
"What?" said Karen.
"The dead Stone, darling. He wore sharp suits like this." (His father had all the albums and pics of the early days).
"Mmm, very - " Karen searched for the style.
"Age Concern. For men." He struck the pose.
"Watch out Calvin Klein."

"For quality and value and, let's face it Kaz, good old fashioned service, Oxfam and co leave the competition standing."

"Lovely old girls down Shaftesbury's," I agreed, not that I'd be seen dead in their clothes, but I bought Mum a teapot once.

"And they really don't mind you lifting a few things at the same time." Trust McEwan.

"You don't, do you - ?" Karen was outraged.

"Just kidding, Kaz."

She didn't believe him, but she giggled. Noone ever called her Kaz except McEwan.

McEwan looked at the mad cows in the fields, munching grass and staring. "How can anyone eat a cow?"

"Oh God, you're not an animal liberationist as well, are you?" said Karen.

"Me? I am...an ...ANIMAL..." he roared. "And we animals will inherit the earth. We will eat...PEOPLE. Grrrr."

He roared and clawed at us. The little girl sitting with her mum at the next table laughed and laughed at him. McEwan loved her appreciation and suddenly turned and roared at <u>her</u>, scaring her badly and making her cry. Her mum cuddled her.

"I'm really really sorry," said McEwan, ashamed. "I'm just a boy. Honest. Look."

When the mum and the girl got off, she looked round at him, frowning, and he lifted his lip and growled, very softly, and she almost smiled.

Suddenly we could see the sea, grey and misty.

"I want to see The Lanes," said Karen. "They were in Time Out. Loads of posh clothes shops."

I wanted to do the pier. I'd seen Quadrophenia. McEwan wanted to do the Aquarium which he remembered visiting when he was little and got scared down in the dark dungeons. Sea monsters, pin ball machines or chic clothes? The only thing we agreed was that we'd meet on the pier, have fish and chips, a few beers, then do one of Brighton's very best clubs. Karen had seen them in Time Out.

McEwan screamed and said:

"Fuck your posh shops. I'm going to eyeball the big fish," and he went off to ask a crowd of foreign kids the way to the Aquarium.

"He's gone!" said Karen in a triumphant whisper and pulled me away, running into Brighton.

Yes! Karen all to myself. Young love in the lanes in the rain.

On the pier Karen paid a fortune to have her palm read by Sister Amelia in a blue hut while I watched the sea swelling underneath. When she came out she looked like she'd been crying.

"You alright?"

She laughed and sobbed. "I'm going to have four children and two men. Be very very happy and travel faraway."

She leaned on me and I put my arm round her. We walked slowly along the wet deck, getting blown about.

"So what's the problem?" I said, cheerily.

"I don't want four bloody children and two men," she said through her sobs and laughs. "I'm not even sure I want to be very very happy. I want more than that."

"Candy floss?"

"I <u>hate</u> candy floss. It sticks to you."

She hugged me tight and we walked on down the pier.

"McEwan's pretty manic today, isn't he?" she said.

"Don't worry, he's used to it."

She put her arm through mine. The pier was wet and empty.

"You're so different you two. Why are you mates?"

"Dunno. He's a good scally."

"There are three types of men." She had a theory. "Mad scallies like McEwan. Bastards like Ian. And the unfathomable ones like you."

"I'm just so shallow you think there's got to be more to me but there ain't."

She squeezed my arm and pulled me closer. I loved her clinging on to me, so tight and warm I could hardly listen to what she was saying, just smiled dumbly at the charming people on the pier.

"So how's Ian?" I asked casually as possible.

"No idea. I'm through with him. He's probably found himself another young playmate on a number 2 bus by now."

"Yes!" Fisting the sky. "Why?"

"We had a fight."

"What sort of fight?"

"Don't ask me about it, OK? It's over."

"Did he hurt you?" I wanted to know.

"I slapped him and he slapped me back rather hard, that's all. He cut my ear." She pulled back her hair to show me where her earring had ripped.

"The bastard."

"Don't worry about it, Alex. It's over. I won't see him again."

And that was that. I felt like the kid who wouldn't understand. Again. But this time it was sweet, very sweet. And we went on, arms tight round each other.

The fairy lights were reflecting all over the wet deck. Magic. We leaned over the rail and watched the deep dark sea swaying and crashing. She said:

"Do you ever get a really strong desire to jump in and just disappear?"

"Yeah, like a dare."

"But you know you're never going to do it."

"Yeah. But like you could if – "

Someone suddenly shoved us up against the rail then grabbed us and held us. Karen screamed. McEwan was playing scary games. I coulda slapped him.

"You twat," I spat.

"Just piss off, McEwan," said Karen, walking off, sick of him.

He was looking strange and dishevelled.

"I've been done over," he said quietly. "All my money. All my gear."

He said he'd been conned by a group of Italian kids who somehow got his dosh, draw and trainers. What? He couldn't explain.
"Have you told the police?" said Karen.
"Don't be dumb," he said. "Let's go home."
"Fuckinell," I said. "The night's just beginning."
"Yeah and I've just been attacked, mate. I'm fucking soaked and I got no shoes."
Shivering in his shiny wet dead Stone suit. End of Brighton pier.

On the train home he put his dirty bare white feet on the next seat, pulled his legs up tight and crashed out, hugging himself where his cuts were, up his arms, to keep warm. I still hadn't told Karen about his cuts and burns, cos it was a secret, wasn't it? He'd showed me, his mate, and it was personal, between me and him. So personal, I had to forget it.

She put her head on my shoulder and whispered:
"I don't want to go out with him ever again."
When McEwan woke up, he said:
"Thanks for letting me come with you. Sorry I fucked up."
He tried to smile that stupid smile. I felt embarrassed for him, didn't know what to say.

GUNS OF BRIXTON

Karen was so excited cos she was about to finish her job and go home to Bath before her Moroccan trek. Karen in Marakesh, so romantic, so daring. But me I was sick, sick she was leaving, a bit sick she never asked me, did she? But then she had told me, hadn't she, that Ian was a fat violent bastard who she won't be seeing again. But she will be seeing me, won't she? Oh yes. Especially after tonight.

Tonight at the Fridge, all night, we both wore white and glowed in the dark, dazzled each other, laughing alot, very hot. She held me tight and really kissed me.
"I'm really going to miss you," she said, looking deep into my eyes. "And Brixton."
She kissed me hard again. I believed her. She danced like an angel. And we danced like hell together, really happy, and I got that feeling you get when the dance takes over, when you don't know what you're doing but you can't go wrong, everything fits, your brain, your body and you and everyone else dancing. Fucking perfect. Nowamin?

Mango juice in the morning from the shop up the hill. And a bag of doughnuts, sweet and sticky. She had to go into work, Saturday morning. Just time to go to her flat and have fast sex for the first time ever. She didn't say why. Who cares? She squeezed both her hands down the front of my jeans and watched my reaction. Then she pulled my old belt and buttons and yanked my jeans and FCUKs down to my feet and I did hers even faster and we rolled onto the floor. I couldn't believe it, this is sex with Karen, on the floor, for real. Kissing and licking. Stroking and poking. Pushing and shoving. Shooting and shouting. FUCK! Thanks. Bloody ell. Yeah, she said, come and have a shower. Fucking power shower! I gelled her all over and we started all over again, in the shower. Body Shop gel, totally natural and not tested on wild animals. FUCK! Then she had to go.

Outside in the sunshine, I didn't want to leave Brixton. Where Karen lives. I lay down on the grass by the Mass church. A drunk stinker sat down beside me and asked me for 20p for the bus home and I gave him a pound and he said bless ya mate and I stretched out and fell asleep with a big smile on my face, safe and warm, totally in love with Karen.

That was the day a man got shot dead by the police in Brixton cos he had a cigarette lighter like a gun. I heard the cop cars screaming around.

That night, me Mum asked me if I'd heard about it. "I was in Brixton when it happened," I said, just to shock her.
"For God's sake be careful, Alex. It's like Miami Vice round here sometimes".
She hated it. She started a petition against Electrical Heaven, the shop on the High Road that

sells tellies and kettles and toasters – and guns. She said: "I went in there today and threatened him. He said they're only air pistols and replicas. I said they look pretty real to me. You can't stop me, he said. Why not do us a favour, I said, make us all feel safer, dump the guns. Sorry, love, he said, it's my business. And it's our community, I said. God I was angry. Gun shops, death-wish cigarette lighters. It's crazy."

"Talking of er death wishes," I said, casual as hell. "Why do some kids cut themselves? You know, like a habit."
McEwan's cuts had got into my brain. She looked at me, wondering why I was asking, then just told me.
"A girl at the unit told me it was the only thing that relieved the pain and confusion. And it was real, something she could show."
She stopped and watched me listening.
"Why are you asking, darling? Not thinking of it, are you? "
"Oh yeah."
"McEwan?"
"Nah. Just someone at college. They said that boys don't do it. You know."
"Course they do. Not so much but…sure you're OK, love?"
"Mum. I'm on top of the world."

I was an all. In fact, I really wanted to tell her right then that I just had sex with Karen today, twice, once on the floor, once in the shower. But you can't, can you? You can't talk about girls and sex, the pain and passion. Not to your mum. So who the fuck <u>do</u> you tell? Who gives a toss anyway? Only you.

I played "Guns of Brixton" and "Death or Glory" from Dad's old Clash album. Bad day for the Brixton man, great day for me, cos me, I'm alive, and not only that, mate, I'm fucking Karen, aren't I?

TALENT

I didn't want to see McEwan. I didn't want him and his dramas ruining my little love story. I hadn't talked to him since the Brighton disaster and he hadn't reappeared at College after Easter. Then he called me, up high and active again, risen from the depths and plotting his great escape from Lambeth College, Streatham and England.

They wrote and told him he could repeat the whole AS year, change to IT and DTP, or leave ASAP. No one had noticed he'd already scarpered. Now all he badly needed was money to split the country and seek asylum somewhere dark and exotic.

The fact that he wanted a job shocked and pleased his anxious parents. His father even got a business friend to concoct a reference for him. With no qualifications, he had to convince people of his natural talents of which he had many but no proof. No problem. He landed a job as a luggage porter working long hours in a huge hotel for excited tourists and bored businessmen.

He was soon making massive profits, using his charm and cheek to cadge big tips from tourists for shifting their bags.
"It's fucking simple, Alex. Sometimes I look down at my scruffy shoes, like Oliver Twist, sweet and umble like, and just wait. And sometimes I look them straight up and ask for a nice big note, please. They can't refuse."

He had a green uniform with gold buttons and smiled appealingly all day long. He even got friendly with a receptionist girl who turned out to be shagging the hotel manager. He was bitter about that, but continued smiling for the money.

Back at the college, I was being interviewed for target-setting by my personal tutor who picked on my talent for choosing bad friends. McEwan was a very persuasive boy, she said, but he's gone now. So what did I want to do with my life? If I wanted to go to university or a good job with a big company, she said, I needed to buckle down. What you do now affects your life forever.
Fuckinell, Miss.

But I wasn't worried, not me. I knew I'd do alright and me Mum would be proud of me. But when she came to the college open evening the only thing she remembered was the teachers' great relief that McEwan was no longer there to drag me down further into delinquency and cynicism. She always got dramatic after parents' evenings. When we got home, she attacked me for allowing myself to be corrupted by McEwan.
"Why did you go along with him?"
"It wasn't like what they're saying, Mum. Honest. He wasn't even there most of the time. They just hated him cos he questioned them, that's all."
"And look where all his questioning's got him."
"He's doing alright. He's earning a packet and he's going to travel the world."

"And when he's finished bumming around what's he gonna be? A hotel porter? Drug dealer?"
That was just crap and I shouted at her:
"Who cares? It's his life isn't it? You can't control him. Or me, for that matter. We're not like your troubled kids, remember. But you care more about them, don't you, because they're <u>sick</u>. Sick and hopeless."
She shouted back.
"Listen, Alex. I care about those kids so I can earn the money for you and me, alright? There's no one else, remember. So when you go to university – "
"I'm not going to university. I'll get a job."
"OK. Forget it. Waste your life then."
End of argument. Both saying things we didn't mean.

Later, of course, she came and did one of her touching sorry-but-I'm-your-mum speeches.
"I'm really proud of you, love, but I don't say it enough. I care more about you than anyone else in the world and that's why I want you to do well. I'm your mum. So I worry. And I don't want you to be a pointless rebel like your father and chuck your life away."
"Don't worry about it, Mum. I'm not like my Dad. Or Paul McEwan. OK?"
"Yeah, OK." She kissed the top of my hair. "You're right. You've got to do it your way. That Mr Morrison said you're a talented boy. I liked him alot."
Shit, did she fancy him?

"He's married." I said quickly. "Two sweet kids. Er how's Matt?"

"I'm sure he's just fine. I haven't seen him for a while and don't intend to."

She smiled. I understood. She said:

"And how's your Karen? She's always so friendly on the phone."

"Yeah, she's good. She's going to Morocco soon."

"And leaving you behind?"

I nodded and looked tragic.

"But hey!" she shouted, joyful. "We're going to the dales in August with Grannie and Granpa!" She pulled a desperate, apologetic face. "You are coming, aren't you, love?"

I suddenly, badly, passionately wanted to be in the scorching heat of Morocco, smoking a blaster spliff with Karen under the African stars.

"Yeah. I'm coming."

PASSION

So. Back to the love story. Karen's dumped her old lover, we've had sex at last, and life has a warm glow, doesn't it?

Yes, the sun was shining on Streatham and little Alex was beaming. But you know how it is just when everything feels perfect, you get this creepy feeling it ain't real? When I called Karen a couple of days later, she sounded pissed off, nothing much to say. Period perhaps, tired, I dunno, but I got this feeling that Karen was troubled. She called me back the next day to apologise, sweet and friendly. She'd been stressed out, she said, she'd explain when we met. What?

I was gonna meet her at Cicero's hippy café on Clapham Common after college, and I just wanted everything to be perfect again. I'd been feeling so fucking good about me and Karen after The Fridge and sex on the floor and in the shower that Saturday morning in sunny Brixton. I wanted to be excited about seeing her again, but I was nervous.

You can sit outside at Cicero's, watching the grungy kids smash up the scruffy old toys, and the cars race through the common. She was sitting there already, staring at nothing. She hugged me and said have some cake. Passion cake, she said. I can't remember what it tasted like, just remember the passion bit, catching her eye. She looked embarrassed, sweet. She hardly ate any, had a fag instead, unusual for her except at night.

I think I was telling her one of McEwan's hotel stories when she stopped me and said:
"Sorry Alex. I'm hopeless at this."
"What?"
"I've got to tell you. Ian's moving in with me."
That was all she said. At first I thought oh shit, then I realised what she was saying. He's moving in with her. Big time. Real shit. Not passion cake. This was serious, like he's moving in with me and I won't be seeing <u>you</u>, mate. I was totally gobsmacked. She kept looking at me with this stupid worried sad look. I said:
"You said he was a bastard. And he <u>hurt</u> you."
"I know. But he's come back. He's left his family. We're going to see how it goes, you know? It's complicated, Alex."
"Yeah?" I didn't believe her, I didn't understand, and the way she told me was like she was explaining it to a kid, me.
"I still want to see you, you know," she said.
"That's gonna be hard, isn't it?"
"Ian can't dance."
"Exactly."
She tried to smile. I coulda hit her. I looked around. A couple of kids were fighting over a giant snail on wheels.
"We just had sex, for fuck's sake."
"Yeah, it was really good. I – "
"So?"
"So - there's more to it than that, Alex."

I couldn't look at her. There was nothing to say. I'd lost her. I was going to leave. She said:

"You mean a lot to me, you know."

I kept hitting my lighter on the table and she put her hand on mine to stop me and hold me but I pulled my hand away.

"Alex," she said, like I shouldn't be upset, like I was a hurt little boy.

When I got up to go she got up too. Half the passion cake was left. Walking back across the common to the shops and bustops, she said:

"This may sound crazy, but Ian's gonna be in the flat by himself when I go to Morocco and Celia and Ho are in the States all summer. He's writing a maths book for toddlers, to make loads of money, and Celia's gonna do the graphics. So if you want go for a drink or if you need a place to crash out, he's there."

"Are you serious?"

"Yeah. He likes you."

But I hated him. Didn't she see that?

We stopped at the High Street. I didn't want her to go. She kissed me, a little kiss, and squeezed my arm. She went left and I went right.

How dare she ditch me? I didn't understand. I didn't believe her. I sort of hated her, but I didn't really, I wanted her. So what do I do now then? Go and get mashed? Drown myself?

Nah. I walked all the way home and watched telly with me Mum, a double Friends repeat, the ones

where Chandler and Monica think they're having a secret affair and everyone actually knows but no-one says. I wasn't really watching, I knew it all. Mum ruffled my hair.
"You allright love?"
"Yup."

I couldn't believe it. It was all fucking over.

EXCITED

May. Exam fever. It was getting hotter. Nipples and navels were flashing through linen, silk, cotton and polyester. Top colours were strong this summer. Shocking pink, egg yellow, ultra violet and black. How could I concentrate? I couldn't work at home, Chilli Peppers full on, gawping at girls out the window, downstairs' cat stalking two blue tits and a robin red-breast in the pear tree. No chance. I had to shift.

Since Karen ditched me I was edgy and excited, like something else had to happen, good or bad. I was completely mixed up. I wanted her, missed her, and hated her. It hurt. I wanted something else.

I went into the library determined to put all my grief behind me and be an AS success. Two smart girls looked at me and my heart leapt. I sat down and looked cool, got my big sociology books out. Is the family a universal institution? I was going to nail it. When my phone bleeped, everyone looked and the librarian took the opportunity to remind all students that mobiles must be turned off at all times in the library. Sorry, I mouthed to her, gave her a big smile and went outside.

It was McEwan texting me. I hadn't seen him since Brighton at Easter, what with me exams and him working non-stop at the hotel. He didn't know Karen and me were like dead.

Message was: *US spies in stretm xcape to clapm NOW.* What? He was so bad at text.

I called him. He'd finished his hotel shift and was drinking outside The Sun at Clapham Common.
"It's a beautiful day and I made some massive tips," he said. "Come and celebrate with Maria and Lala and me."
"Who?"
"Exotic chambermaids, mate."
Fuck the family. I ran to the tube, pretty excited.

McEwan was on the edge of a table outside The Sun laying it off to two stunning long-black-haired brown girls. Bloody ell. He introduced me to Maria and Lala and we shook hands, so polite. Long soft hands.
"They come from a beautiful island in the Philippines and now they work in the Strand Palace Hotel making beds and cleaning toilets."
They smiled. What do you say?
"Er, you like the hotel?" I asked.
"Oh yes," they said.
"And London?"
"Oh yes. London is special."
"But sadly they have to leave us now," said McEwan, tenderly touching one girl's hand. "I just wanted them to meet you first. We're all going to have a picnic on Wimbledon Common and you're invited, mate."
"Thank you. You like picnics?" I said to the chambermaids.

"Oh yes. And Wimbledon tennis men."
They giggled and we all stood up and shook hands again. McEwan kissed the one with whom he was clearly developing a top-seed doubles act and they left, looking back and waving to us, how sweet.
"What do you think of them then?" he was keen to know.
"Tropical island sunshine. Malibu on legs," I oozed.
"What about your one? Lala."
"This is a set-up isn't it?"
"They go everywhere together, those two."
"So I amuse Lala while you shag the legs off Maria - ?"
He nodded, waggled his tongue and blinked, fast and filthy.

He brought two mega glasses of that weird white Belgian beer with a lemon stuck in it. He had money now.
"I wasn't kidding about those spies in Streatham, mate. It was in the local paper. Explains those weird black kite manoeuvres on the common lately. No one holding the strings." He tapped his nose, in the know, eyes-wide and fingers pointing.
He was in a very buzzy mood, wasn't he? This hotel-portering lark had lightened him up nicely. Filipino girls, picnics and giant white beers. No more sick cuts and burns, please. He can't still be doing that crap, can he? I didn't wanna know. Cos this was my old mad McEwan, my mate, grinning and gushing, just like before, larking about while I

sweat over essays on fucking cross-cultural institutional intimate social groupings and suffering severe heart-break at the same time. I had to tell him about Karen, didn't I? About her dumping me and me being badly, tragically fucked off. He, big boy, gripped my shoulder and said, don't worry mate, let her go, I'll sort ya. And he told me about how he sorted this German businessman at his hotel.

"He's going out for the evening, right, and asks me: where can I find a girl? You know what I want, he says and gives me a look like he means business, sex business. Fuck, I think, Soho? a phone box? I dunno. Then he says, a bar is OK, but a bar where I can meet a girl, you understand? Oh, I say, in that case try Stringfellows, St Martin's Lane. Or the place opposite. And I get him a taxi, he gives me a fiver and off he goes."
"So what's the place opposite?" I asked him, impressed with his knowledge of London's sex hot spots.
"It's a fucking hair salon. Anyway, today he comes up and says: Thank you, thank you, sir - it was a very good night. And he shakes my hand and slips me twenty quid! Twenty fucking quid. Stringfellows? I ask him. No, he says, the place opposite!"

"Yeah!" I slapped McEwan on the back. "Top geezer for sex tips!"
"That's me, mate. I'll see you right." He punched me on the shoulder, like good old mates do. "Stick

with me, Alex boy, and that Kaz girl will dissolve into… thin… air."

"Don't even mention her," I said and waved her memory away into the big white clouds floating over The Sun.

We went on to the common for some freedom, Red Stripe and smoke. It smelt strong in the fresh air. We sucked hard, hadn't shared a spliff since the troubled kids' party. Nice out there, it was, under a big tree, traffic in the distance, birds close. You could hear yourself breathe. We just watched. A girl was moving slowly across the horizon, head up and hair blowing, with a big dog flapping about her. McEwan said something stupid about woofers or woollies or something and I started giggling, couldn't stop, and he must've thought he was being really hilarious cos he told me another sexy hotel story to keep me hooting me pants off.

"Listen to this one, Alex," he said, chuckling already. "Anthony, he's the head porter, says: room 521, Mac, the African Queen has asked for you personally. You'll be alright there, mate, he says and gives me a wink. So off I go up to this woman's room, fifth floor, right?"

He stood up to represent racing up to the fifth floor, really keen.

"I knock on her door – " he went and thumped the tree trunk, one two three

" – and she takes her time coming, yeah, and when she opens up she looks like she's just come out the shower, she's in this gorgeous red silk dressing gown with a white towel wrapped round her head. She was a queen alright, man, a beautiful big African queen, and I was her boy servant, no argument. She says, you like humping? Like <u>what</u>? I say. You are the baggage boy? she says. Oh yeah. So now you hump <u>me</u>, yes? I pay you a big tip, she says. Oh yes, big tip, anything, madam. Alex, I was shitting myself, man, she coulda swallowed me up, you know? And she gives me one of those red condoms with knobs on. Oh my God, I'm in a flap, can't open the pack, can't get the fucking hood on – "

He was replaying his whole sexy hotel drama, there in the middle of Clapham Common, and I watched, gobsmacked but not giggling any more. So he tried even harder.

"She goes over to the window and opens it, right, holds onto the safety bar and leans through the net curtains to watch the street below. Then she sticks her arse out and pulls up her gown. Great big arse, man. Come on, boy, she says, ma little pussy's waiting. And in I go, easy. And we're rocking, you know? Over the fucking Strand!"

Course now, McEwan had his arms round the tree trunk, didn't he, and he was shagging the fucking tree, shocking Clapham, how common.

"And then she starts going: red buses, The Strand, red buses, The Savoy, black cabs, Simpsons, black cabs, Soho, Soho, oh, London, London oh oh OH! She's too fast for me, mate. She shoves me off with her arse, pulls the johnny off me and chucks it, squeezes my cheek and goes: I am <u>so</u> excited, dear, London <u>so</u> excites me, you know. You like jazz? Come and hear me sing tonight, baggage boy. And she gives me two tickets for Ronnie Scott's and a £10 tip. Jazz Queen from Jo'burg. Tell all your friends about me, honey. Certainly will, madam. When I get downstairs, Anthony says: so how many tickets did <u>you</u> get, Mac? Leroy got four!"

End of performance. He held out his hands and bowed. It was all a load of kak, of course. Some sad old porter's porn story.

"Well lucky Leroy," I said.

"What?" he screamed. "Is that all you can say? Lucky Leroy? Well fuck you, Alex. You don't believe me, do ya? You don't believe me!"

I started giggling again. What a tosser.

"You bastard! It's true. Believe me! You wanka, Alex. I'll make you fucking believe me."

Suddenly he pulled me off my log and onto the grass, tickling me hard. I was choking and pissing myself. I hit him and kicked him, but he sat on me and held my wrists so I couldn't move, I gave up.

"Believe me?"

"Piss off."

He twisted my wrists and forced his forehead against mine.

"Believe me now?"

I gave in.

"Yeah, yeah. I believe ya. African Queen. Big arse. Big tip. True story. OK?"

"Yeah. Right."

He got off me. I sat up, pulled the leaves and twigs and shit out of my hair, then looked up to see him leaping, fisting the sky, totally mental. The winner.

I sprayed my beer over him like Schumacher does and raced for the Angel of Temperance, with McEwan chasing and cussing me and laughing like crazy.

We're heading for Brixton and music and we dip into some crushed cool bar on Clapham High Street. After a fast beer and a headful of screaming chat, I hate the place and walk out with someone's bottle of Sol and a Tesco bag. McEwan can't believe I've done it. I shove the Tesco bag into my own bag and wait till we're deep into the back streets of Brixton.

There's a make-up bag, two packs of fags, a purse with £20 and a phone. Just as we're looking, the fucking phone rings, a very irritating ring. Bold, I answer it fast. A loud girl is screaming:
"Have you nicked my phone?"
"Yeah sorry."
"You fucking thief. You bastard. You - you there?"
"Yeah."
"Who are you?"
"Not telling."
McEwan's watching, eyes wide, impressed, hysterical.
"Look mate, I want my fucking phone back," demands the girl.
"Sure. Where are you?"
"Where you fucking nicked it. The Fine fucking Line. Clapham fucking High Street."

"OK. Look - I'll leave it all wrapped up in the bag in a skip in Baytree Road in Brixton. Baytree Road. Got that?"

"In a skip? In fucking Brixton?"

"What's wrong with Brixton?"

"It's fucking miles away."

"It's not. Anyway, nice to talk," and I cut the call.

"Not a pleasant girl," I say to McEwan who's still gobsmacked by my nerve.

We confiscate her Marlboro Lights cos they're bad for her, then I chuck the bag into the skip.

"You is crazy man," says McEwan.

My heart's thumping. I need to get moving, lose myself in the crowd.

And so we surge into Mass where the rhythms are rolling in every room and we leap and jerk to the jungle, drum and bass. Tonight is Mishmash and we're right in it, the crowd disturbance, the soft mosh pit mayhem, the ecstasy and excitement, all night long. It feels right to be with McEwan, just him and me, rolling again, with nothing about Karen, not a thought, not tonight.

Outside, it felt cold. We were hot. Our clothes were wet. What can you say?

"Good night, mate."

"Fuckin good night."

PAIN

Course, it didn't go away, did it? The pain, that is. I couldn't stand it. I wanted someone else to feel it. Preferably Ian. He's the bastard who gets kicked out by his wife who can't take any more, so he dumps himself on Karen cos Karen's a soft touch and scared cos he hurt her before, I saw the evidence. I couldn't really hate Karen, but I wanted to make <u>him</u> pay. I didn't know <u>how</u> yet but I'd think of something. And I was going to ask McEwan to help.

This was when I really wanted to trust McEwan. That was a fucking good session with him at Mass. The smokes on the common, his African queen, the fight, nicking the Nokia. Brilliant. Just me and him, blagging and screaming, like before. Now I needed him to be a best mate and do my plan. I wanted to humiliate Ian.

We met by the bandstand with a couple of cans. But McEwan didn't get my trials and tribulations, did he? He said:
"Quit vexing about him. He's not the problem, she is. She's the slag, mate."
"Fuck off." I could have hit him, but I needed his help. So I laid it on. "Listen - he's got a family, a poor little family, up there in Liverpool, depending on him. It's adult time, man. He should be at home with the wife and kids, not shacking up with a girl half his age in Brixton. He needs a good beating, like he beat up Karen."

But he didn't get my passion, my hurt pride, my pain. Let's face it, McEwan was pretty clueless on the personal side of life. Big on global disasters, shit at the personal. Personal was a joke. Just listen to this. He said:

"I shagged her too, you know."

"Who?"

"Karen."

"You what? You shagged Karen?" I stood up.

"Yeah."

"You didn't."

"Yeah. Like I didn't want to tell you before – "

"I don't believe you. You said she's not pretty."

"But she's a nice shag."

I went mad. I pulled him up and punched him, hard in the belly, and he bent over, coughing and laughing, on his knees.

"Sorry mate…didn't think…you'd mind…" he choked.

"Fuck off will ya?"

He looked up at me, his ex-mate, and gasped out:

"Alex. It was…a joke, right? I thought you'd…appreciate it."

He was screwing me up. I held his arms tight and looked him straight in the eyes.

"Tell me the truth, McEwan, for fuck's sake."

"I just have."

"Did you shag Karen?"

"Read my lips. I did not have sexual relations with that woman."

"You bastard."

Well did he? Course not. And she wouldn't, would she? No. Not with him. But that sort of thing really gets me. Specially from your best mate. Best mate? What? Yeah, a best mate who shows me his wounds, needs me, trusts me, then kicks me. That hurt.

Back home, I hadn't told Mum about Karen yet, it was too painful, but she probably knew somehow, she usually did. When I told her my head was aching and all down my neck, she got her Body Shop oil, sat me down, pulled my T-shirt off, stood behind me and massaged my shoulders, neck and head. Pain relief. Her hands were strong; she hadn't massaged me since I was a kid, but she knew exactly what to do.

You know how some men - like Ian and Matt for instance – go on about how they just don't understand women, don't trust them, they're a complete mystery, mate? I never thought that before all this. Like, me Mum knew what she was doing and I trusted her. She'd stick up for me. But that's mothers, I suppose, and they're different to girls. With Karen, it sounds sad now but I really thought I knew her, knew how she thought, and I always thought she'd choose me in the end. So when she told me in Brighton that Ian was a bastard, I was well pleased but not surprised, only to be expected. But then when she tells me a coupla weeks later that Ian's moving in with her, I was gobsmacked dumb. Suddenly I didn't understand her. She was, like they said, a complete fucking mystery. I didn't blame her but I didn't trust her either, and I didn't want to see her again.

Ian of course was a different matter. I definitely wanted to see <u>him</u> again, on his own, to teach him a private lesson. But McEwan wasn't interested, he respected Ian too much. So I had to deal with the fat bastard myself, didn't I?

McEwan said what I really needed was company, nice new girls, like Lala and Maria. He'd sort it, he said, but remember, mine's Maria. Oh yeah? Like I said, he wasn't strong on the personal but he was trying.

I woke up in the night, thinking about everything, had to put the radio on to block my brain. *Kiss FM* to make it all feel better. The pain, that is. But it didn't.

WIMBLEDON COMMON

This was the picnic with the Filipino chambermaids, thoughtfully arranged by McEwan so I could forget about Karen and he could snog Maria in the bushes. My girl Lala was sweet and fit, no doubt about that, but what exactly can you expect on Wimbledon Common with two exotic chambermaids and a wild boy on a cloudy Sunday in June? Well. This is what happened.

McEwan brought them along after their morning hotel shift and we met in an old posh pub in Wimbledon. They were both wearing white, on the look out for international tennis stars. Wimbledon Common is deep common compared to Streatham or Clapham; we walked for miles into the dark interior and set up camp in a secret dip. They waved out a big white sheet to catch the crumbs and keep their skirts clean. McEwan brought a small music machine and his *Roots Manuva* CDs, wearing dark shades and a green T shirt. So cool. I don't think so.

These girls had a bag full of Filipino specialities they'd made, everything wrapped in foil like your mum would. Brilliant spicy meat sticks and chicken legs and giant prawns and rice in leaves. I took Pringles and beer. McEwan had already glugged most of a bottle of wine. He had two. Maria and Lala preferred Evian and when they smoked they looked naughty.

Maria was 19 and Lala was 18. An agency had recruited them to work here for a year, London hotels being desperate for cheap chambermaids. They were making lots of money to buy FCUK and Man United labels for their brothers and sisters and urgent medical care for their grandmothers. All on the UK minimum wage. McEwan exploded.

"Bastards! Rich fucking multinational hotel bastards."

He stood up and reached out, bottle in his hand, and spoke for us, the common people, against all the rich bastards and global capitalists who exploit poor Filipino chambermaids, their brothers and sisters and grannies, McEwan and me, and all the common people of the world. He'd asked me to go to this year's May Day riot but I don't wanna associate with all dem clowns on stilts and urban warriors in scary masks, do I? He was on hotel duty on May Day and badly wanted the money so he did his shift then turned into a masked urban guerrilla for the evening. Anyway, here on Wimbledon Common, faraway from the mad city, I clapped and fisted my solidarity and sang the May Day anthem with him.

"Underground, overground, wombling free, the Wombles of Wimbledon Common are we."

We struck hands and chuckled. The girls looked at us like "what?" A bouncy big labrador came sniffing around our patch and McEwan made it jump for some Filipino delicacies.

"Do chambermaids get tips?" I asked.

"Sometimes," they said and giggled. "The old men."

"Do they try to er - ?"

"Fuck you," McEwan helped me out.

The girls screamed.

"Some men ask to take us to bars and restaurants but they are so old and - you know - " they made sick faces and laughed.

"But me and Alex are different, aren't we?" McEwan smiled and stroked Maria's hair, smooth and seductive.

"Oh yes," they giggled. "You are different. You are funny."

McEwan was into his second bottle of wine and getting mashed all by himself. He kissed Maria, like mad and deeply, but she pulled out of rolling over and over into the jungle ferns.

"No! My clothes. They will be green." She stayed firmly on the sheet.

"I adore green clothes," McEwan cried. "Anyway, who cares about clothes

when... when...love yes love calls?"

"What? What is this love? Not me, thank you." Maria was pretty smart.

McEwan waved her away dramatically and lit up a spliff. Lala and I exchanged a neat, knowing look. She had great brown eyes. I was still nervous but getting excited. I took some hits of smoke, showed Lala how, and lay down closer to her.

Other picnickers and Sunday lovers, dogs and common people were drifting home on the horizon. McEwan turns up the volume on Rodney Smith doing *Witness the Fitness*. He starts dancing, pissed and happy to groove on his own for a while. Then he comes to Maria and raves in waves all around her then starts pulling her up.

"Let's dance. Please please please dance with me."

"No, no. I don't like this music," she says.

But he still pulls her up and holds on to her arms, moving her around like a doll.

"Come on baby," he sings to her. "*You set fire to my soul. I'm gonna lose control.*"

Lala and I laugh but Maria is dead serious. He's swinging her around and she's telling him to stop but he doesn't stop, he won't let go, he's dragging her round and round, she's looking desperate and I shout, "Leave it, McEwan." And he suddenly lets go of her and of course she goes sprawling across the grass and McEwan's laughing and falling on top of her and he starts groping, hands up her skirt and top and she struggles free and hits him, then stands up and kicks him in the back, shouting at him. He gets up, still laughing, and she goes and screams right in his face, and he slaps her, once, very hard, in the mouth and knocks her right over. Lala screams and we leap up. Maria's on her knees, panting and sobbing, there's blood on her face. Lala wipes her face, talks in Filipino, comforting and angry, saying her name alot. McEwan's hanging about, trying to be concerned, mumbling things. Lala glares at him.

"Piss off," I tell him but he stays.

"Why didn't she wanna dance?" he says.

"You are a bad man," Lala shouts at him. "You do not do this to girls."

"She hit me first," McEwan goes, pathetic boy.

"Look, just fuck off, will ya?" I tell him hard as I can and he goes off, walking round and round the hollow, stopping to reassure a worried dog-walker that everything's fine, just a little accident.

Maria's mouth is cut and her nose is bleeding. She's gone quiet, letting Lala look after her.

"We go to the police," Lala says to me. "First we go to the hospital and then to the police. Alex, you come with us please."

Oh God. This could get awkward. I can't grass on me mate, can I? No. Even if he has smashed a girl in the mouth. Fuckinell no.

I looked at the damage more closely. Her nose wasn't bleeding much, her lip was cut and swollen. I badly wanted her to be OK.

"She'll be allright," I said like I knew.

"You take us to the hospital," Lala said again.

"I'll get a taxi for you," I said.

"You come to the police with us."

"Let's go and get a taxi."

I went over to McEwan who was swigging wine and muttering.

"You got a tenner? Twenty?"

"What for?"

"They need a taxi and you're paying for it."

He sneered, swayed, pulled two notes out of his pocket and chucked them on the grass. Today's tips. I picked them up.

"Now just go will ya?" I said. "You've done enough damage."

He looked at me, disgusted, and said: "Not much of a mate, are you?"

He shoved me. So I shoved him back and he lost his balance, being pissed, and fell over.

"Go home, McEwan."

He staggered after me, arms up, and I dodged him and he tripped over again.

We looked at each other. I said:

"Listen. You've hurt a girl and I'm going to sort her out. Now piss off."

Lala runs up and screams at him: "Bad boy. Police for you. Trouble for you. Bad bad boy."

He tried to laugh, coughed and threw up instead. Red wine sick. Lala was disgusted. He gave up and sloped off, heaving, not a pretty sight.

I stuffed the picnic into a bag, rescued McEwan's music machine and left the leftovers for the fucking wombles. Maria was recovering and they began to argue in Filipino, probably about going to the police or not. Maria didn't want to.

"We will go home," she said to me, quietly. She looked sick.

"We tell the hotel tomorrow," said Lala. "And the police."

She wanted McEwan dealt with.

It was a very long walk back to the road, with bursts of angry Filipino. Maria held a handkerchief to her mouth and looked down. There were green grass stains down the back of her white skirt. I felt bad for her. All I could say was:

"I'm very sorry."

And she said, "It's OK."

Lala started cussing McEwan again but Maria told her to shut-up. I stopped a cab and gave Lala McEwan's £20. They said they lived in a horrible hostel in Vauxhall. Bloody ell.

THE WATERSHED

I felt sick after that picnic. Sick about those two girls and sick of Paul McEwan. He says he'll cheer me up, sort me out, then it all ends with girls in tears and me clearing up the mess. And then he tells me I'm not much of a mate. Well, he's no mate of mine either, so basically he can fuck off.

Then the sick boy himself calls me and says sorry, mate, sorry, sorry, sorry. You should be, I tell him. He's flying away in a couple of days, and have I got his music machine? Let's meet, he says, and I say OK, bastard. The last time.

I was keeping clear of Brixton Hill, bad memories, so I met him up his end of Streatham, the cool bar by the common called The Watershed where there's no sign of water. Daft Punk on loud. He was late, swung in, bought a beer and - "Hey Alex, here's my trip!" - started drawing his big journey from Europe to Asia on the table with beer, kicking off on an easyjet to Athens and heading east on boats and trucks through Turkey and Afghanistan to India. He wanted to impress me, but I slid my bottle across the table and trashed it. He was about to shout and I said: "You shouldn't have hit that girl, McEwan. You really hurt her."
He didn't want to know. He said:
"You've just destroyed two continents. I don't know where I'm going now."
"What about Maria? You hit her. Hard."

"Yeah. Shame. End of a beautiful relationship. I had to go and see the Duty Manager today. Lala had told him why Maria wasn't at work. He told me that wasn't the way to treat girls, take it easy, eh? Man to man stuff."

"Listen, mate, you really messed her up. You were....you were totally out of order." I sounded like Phil Mitchell but I was dead serious. "They wanted me to go to the police with them. You coulda been in a load more shit."

"Thanks, bruvver. Appreciate it. I was wrecked actually. Pretty bad." He held out his hand and slapped it hard. "Bad boy. Ouch."

I grabbed his arm and leaned across.

"Listen McEwan. You're always mouthing off about global violence and exploitation and respecting people and all that and then you go and slap up a girl for not letting you grope her. You fucking hurt people too, you know."

I meant it, really meant it. He shut up for a moment, then he said:

"I lost it, didn't I?" Getting real at last. "I do lose it sometimes. I'm doing alright, but there are good days and bad days. And fuck awful days, like yesterday." Then he held up his arms and appealed to the whole bloody bar: "It's how I is, man, it's how I is."

"You're serious, aren't you?"

He's right of course: McEwan will always be McEwan. Half bum, half boy.

"Seriously serious, bruvver. Course I am. Wanna pizza? They're bloody good here. I'll buy ya."

"Nah. I'm meeting someone. A girl."

That was a lie. I couldn't stay with him. I poked at his puddle map. "That's a massive journey, mate."

"Yeah. About fucking time too. Bye-bye Streatham. England. St George." He stood up and did a Henry V, arm stretched out to the A23. "The world!"

"What are you gonna do out there?"

"Man, I is gonna...surf the ocean. Smoke opium. Stop wars. Start a religion. Nowamin. And what wid you, bruvver?"

I put my finger in the spilt beer puddles and drew a straight line through the remains of Europe and Asia and his magical escape route.

"Here's The Watershed and this is me trekking up the High Road. The longest high road in the world. To see a sweet girl on Streatham Hill."

"That's a tough journey, man. And Alex – " he put on his stupid

trust-me face "– forget about Karen. And Ian. Water under the bridge, eh?"

I never listened to his advice and I didn't want to talk about it, so I got up and said well I'm off and he said thanks mate and hugged me hard.

"Listen, mate," he said, most sincere. "No more violence to girls on picnics. I promise."

And that's when he gave me the picture of him as a Hindu god with ten fucking arms: a passport photo stuck on a postcard. What?

I started walking up the longest high road in the world, past the ice rink and the pool. Why did I ever get mixed up with McEwan? Because the others bored me and he was the only boy I knew who hated football and MacDonalds and still made me laugh. But he wasn't funny now. And I was in pain and he couldn't help me. He was, like Karen said, basically a prat.

Past the Odeon, Caesars and Megabowl. A boy sat in the back of a cop car, blood on his face, shocked people around. I was so sick of Streatham. I was sick of everything. I thought about my dad, not that he was any help, but I might as well get totally tragic while I'm at it. So I spoke to him through the High Road din, like I used to when I was 6 or 7.

"I'm seventeen, Dad, and I'm badly pissed off. I'm sick of me mate McEwan and I've been dumped by a girl for an old man and basically I want to teach him a lesson but I don't know what to do and -"

Some girls walked past and giggled at me talking to the traffic. Sad boy. Still, me mum loves me, doesn't she? There's always me mum.

When I got home she was sitting in the gloom listening to a girl folk singer. She put the lamp on; tears in her eyes.

"Don't worry, love, it's just this song about a girl watching over her lover's grave and talking with his ghost. It always gets me." She giggled. "I was just thinking I should go and sit by Sean's stone at the crematorium and see what happens."

I didn't feel like laughing.

"So's how's that Paul McEwan then?"

"The world tour starts tomorrow."

"You're gonna miss him, aren't you love?"

"Nah."

I chucked his mad god-card portrait in the bin then took it out again and stared at it. "To my mate Alex" on the back. What a prick. And I kept it.

FAKE

With McEwan out of the country and Karen out of my life, there was business to see to. As you know, Ian Trogg, her old lover, badly needed a fright. Trogg. I got his surname by calling the South Bank University and acting dumb. Doctor Trogg in fact. Anyway, remember that shop on the High Road that me Mum hated cos it sold toy guns and toasters? Well, I went in. Went in and bought a neat little Colt 25 revolver, £14.50. The grey one was £14, but I preferred the black. Fake, obviously. Only shot yellow pellets.

I knew fuck all about guns, but I knew all about fakes. 60% of guns used in crimes are fakes, you have to be 17 to buy one and you can buy most of them at Electrical Heaven on Streatham High Road. I'd heard the saddoes at school talk guns but it bored me, like they were still on Nintendos or like they thought they were Brixton bad boys, dicing with dying. I wasn't interested then but now, being angry and mad, I needed one.

The Asian shopkeeper said nothing, no awkward questions, but I was prepared in case. "It's for me dad's birthday, mate. He's got all the others."
I came out sweating. I thought everyone on the High Road knew I had a gun. I ran home zig-zagging in case they blasted me. Crazy, eh?

When I got home, I took it out and pointed it at the mirror.

"You're dead, mate."

"No, please – aaah…!"

Kids' stuff. I put it back in the box and tucked it in a drawer me Mum would never open. It's something she really hates, violence. With her, you could do drugs, drink, sex, religion, anything really except guns. But she won't know a thing about it, will she? She'd kill me if she did. But don't worry Mum, this is for one man only. Dr Ian Trogg. And it's a fake, just a laugh. My funny little secret weapon.

But I did tell Lizzie, McEwan's fast-talking cheeky young sister.

She called me and said she had some crap CDs Paul wanted her to return to me.

We met at the cafe on Streatham Common, loads of yellow police signs warning you about vicious attacks and violent robberies. I bought her a Coke and we sat on the grass. She still had the red streaks in her long dark hair that I remembered from the New Year party, cut jeans and knickers showing, very sure of herself. She hated my CDs - old punk stuff McEwan had wanted. She loves Eminem and Streets. Of course.

"I'm playing Eminem and Paul's blasting his Red Records rap and my Dad's like going mad, you know. Course, Paul says Eminem's just white trash acting black and then he gets this South African hip-hop CD which is so good. Even my Mum liked that. She tries to understand Paul and his weird tastes. Poor Mum. He gives her such a hard time."

She took a swig of Coke and said:

"You know when he took that overdose?"

"What overdose? When?"

"At Easter. After he went to Brighton with you. Didn't he tell you?"

"No."

"Oh."

"So?"

"Oh my God. Sorry."

"So – what did he do?"

"He took masses of Mum's pills and vodka. Mum found him on the floor and couldn't wake him up. They rushed him to St George's with Mum's fingers down his throat and his head in a bucket. He was like really out of it. They pumped him out and he came home the next day."

She stopped, looked at me, wide-eyed.

"Didn't he tell you?"

"No," I said, pissed off she knew more than me.

"He coulda died, you know."

I didn't believe her. She exaggerated like her brother. He'd just overdone the skunk and booze, hadn't he, and pumped it for sympathy. Ooo I'm so unhappy, so confused, me. Yeah, good one, McEwan. OK, so he cut himself up a bit, but that was just him pissing about. Bet she didn't know about <u>that</u> and I wasn't going to tell her.

She gabbed on like she can't stop.

"We don't know why he did it. He's changed in the last two years. Like first he got kicked out of St Joseph's, then your college. It was really difficult for Mum and Dad, specially with Dad being a Head Teacher and all that."

"Is he?"

"Yeah, of a girls' school in Croydon." She giggled. "And he's pretty paranoid. He thinks you're to blame, of course."

"What? Me? Why me?" Gobsmacked.

"Cos you're Paul's first best friend and he's gone bad so it must be you."

"That's crap. If your brother's a twat, that's him, not me. Don't blame me."

She laughed at me being sore.

"Hey you're so prickly. Dad doesn't know anything. They're just so stressed out about him, they blame anything except themselves. You got a ciggie?" Quick drag. "He's probably in Rome by now, lucky boy."

"He said he was flying to Athens."

"Well he got as far as Genoa. And there was like some massive demo there against world politicians. We saw it on the telly. One boy got shot dead by the police and Mum nearly had a heart attack thinking it was Paul and just screamed at him when he phoned but Dad said he sounded really happy and hoped he wasn't 'high on something'. He thinks that you and Paul took loads of drugs, you see, and that's how he took the overdose. Did he do lots of drugs?"

"Nah. Bit of this, bit of that."

"I only do spliffs," she said.

And she started telling me about a kids' party where half of them ended up unconscious in St George's or something, but I'd switched off. She blagged on and on like McEwan, must run in the family.

Two little girls were pole-dancing round one of the police signs.

"Don't you get scared walking around Streatham?" she said. "Some of the boys at school are doing self-defence. It's worse for boys, isn't it?"

"Yeah, I've bought a gun for protection. A Colt 25."

"You haven't, have you?"

"Just kidding."

She giggled, relieved, nice joke.

"It's a fake," I said.

She looked confused, worried. She said:

"What do you wanna a fake gun for?"

"I got a plan." So sure and smug.

"You're mad, Alex. You can't act tough, anyone will know you're faking it."

"Fuck off," I said.

And she did. But first she shot me BANG, I collapsed in a heap and she ran. Then she stopped, cupped her hands and screamed FAKE across the common and laughed at me. People looked. I got up quick and went home.

I was still developing my brilliant plan, of course, still working out how to give Ian Trogg a serious fright and then turn it into a joke, a joke with a twist in the blade. Like McEwan when he said he'd shagged Karen, and I nearly killed him, then he goes: just kidding, you twat. You feel stupid, he's in control and it leaves a long sick taste. Only difference is I want Ian Trogg to end up on his knees, well and truly shamed and humbled, and he's saying sorry mate, I got it wrong, you're the one that she wants, she's all yours. And he leaves Karen well alone ever after. Yes!

Well that was the plan.

RESTLESS

August in Streatham, watching bad movies and reading Glue. Me Mum was off work, tidying up and being loud and interactive. I wasn't in the mood.

"You alright, Alex? You're very quiet. Missing your friends?"

She had that sympathetic, knowing look that really got me, like she thought she knew what I was thinking. I hated that.

"We could always do some days out, love. Brighton. Tate Modern. Or -"

"Mum."

She was making me feel like Sadboy of Streatham.

Holidays eh? Hard. We went to Yorkshire for a week with me Grannie and Granpa, in a cottage in a village, Mum and me walking up hills and down dales and driving Grannie and Granpa to beauty spots. Sometimes I stayed in the cottage. So bored, I was chucking dice on the carpet trying for McEwan's ultimate 1x1x1. It can't happen. Two ones yes, but not three. So I gave up and did random options instead, thinking up six brave and crazy deeds for each throw like: shave my hair, suicide, murder, rape. That kind of thing. Just to see what I would have done if I had the nerve.

Then Karen texted me. I didn't see it for days cos mobiles don't work up there. Just said:

"Moroko 2moro Brixton was bril Fanx Alex Weel float take life as it cums PJ Harvey."

Back on Streatham High Road in hot August, only the poor people, the refugees and the Cats Rescue woman were left. I walked around in a sweat, trying hard to take life as it came. I let myself get grabbed by a man outside the Odeon. He had a petition to "Save Our Ice Rink" and stop Tesco bombing it. I signed immediately.
"Bloody multi-nationals destroying our local heritage," I said with feeling and pride. "I mean fuckinell, mate."
The man looked surprised at my passion for protecting ice-skating opportunities in Streatham. I explained:
"Sorry mate, but this means a lot to me, you know, having an ice rink here for kids to learn and get good and – "
Raw emotion. Ice rage.
"That's right, mate," said someone behind me. "You tell em."
I thrust my fist up in solidarity and strode on. I could hear McEwan shouting across Europe:
"Good boy, Alex."

I couldn't think straight. Streatham was stifling. Bloody holidays. Ice rinks. Dice games. Fake guns. Mothers. Fat lovers. I had a MacDonalds and felt sick.

It was me Mum's birthday but I didn't know what the fuck to buy her. In Argos and Oxfam I stood and stared, then staggered into WH Smiths and saw the Buena Vista Social Club CD, reduced to £7.99. Yes! Mum had taken me to the movie a couple of years back and loved it so much she was going to take me to Cuba, but so far she hadn't even bought the CD. So then I found the Rough Guide to Cuba, to show her the way. Yes! Trouble was I didn't have the cash for both. But I did have the nerve. Bold as brass, I bought the Guide then went and slipped the disk in too. No point in mucking about. Didn't even check where the security guard was, so easy, no problem, never been caught, never will. I walked out, smiling to the girl at the till. Yes!

Strolling down the High Road, taking life as it comes, a man suddenly stood in front of me, his hand on my arm, chunky gold rings on his fingers. The WH Smith guard was close up and big. Shit. Big shit.

"Back to the shop, mate."

"Er, why?"

"We want to check your receipt."

"Me Mum paid for it, didn't she?" I said quick as a flash, very convincing.

"And where's she?"

"Behind you."

He just stared at me, like oh yeah, so I screamed "Mum! Mum!" down the road, desperate, people looking. "Mum! Mum!" Then I waved madly like she'd seen me and as he turned slightly to check her out, I jerked free and scarpered fast and smartly down the side roads onto Tooting

Common and into the trees and bushes where the sex girls do business, then round the back-streets to Streatham Hill, the presents down my pants for the CCTV. Mum will be pleased.

Reality hit me walking up our road. Fuck. Can't do that again, no chance, way too close for comfort. I'm on me own now. I've lost McEwan's nerve.

Mum was out, thank God. I gulped two big shots of her gin, straight. Yuk. I felt better. I'd escaped. What a summer, eh? Never known one like it.

Karen's text message had got to me. I kept thinking about her, and about Ian there in her flat, in her bed. I didn't want him there. I wanted her to come home to sunny Brixton and see me, not fucking him. So I can't take life as it comes, Karen, I gotta do something about it.

MY DAY OF POWER

I'd worked it all out in my head. I wanted to scare him, humiliate him and expose him, so Karen could see the <u>truth</u> about Ian Trogg. At least, that's what I had in mind, but I wasn't exactly thinking clearly at this point, being restless and almost arrested, sick about Karen and blaming Ian for absolutely fucking everything. Course I bloody did. I mean, he'd conned her and abused her and upset me. It was obvious I had to give him some grief. Wasn't it?

So this is what I did.

Wednesday morning, September 2001. Me Mum went off early to the troubled kids. I'd had a bad night, must of dreamt about Karen. Whatever. I was in a weird mood and I decided not to do college cos this was the day to take my brand new toy gun out of its box and show Ian. She'd said go and see him, didn't she, give him a break from writing his crap text book. No problem, no fucking problem. I wonder what he does for a laugh on a Wednesday morning in Brixton? Well this one was going to be different.

I walked down Brixton Hill past all those flats with balconies where I could just see me dad doing his balancing act along their narrow ledges. But today it was <u>my</u> act and I didn't care what me dad, me mum, Karen or anyone thought. I knew it was mad without even thinking about it, but I still wanted to do it. I really wanted to trouble him. Hard to explain now, but it felt right then. I put the gun in my pocket and held it tight, on the watch for bad boys, armed robbers and police, tense as hell.

People with orange balloons were waving and singing on the pavement outside a church. DAY OF POWER on the banner. DAY OF POWER on the balloons. Want to hear about the Day of Power, sir? No thanks, I said and nearly pulled the gun out as I waved aside a leaflet, and walked through the crowd. Then, BANG! Christ. A Power balloon burst behind me, and all the Power people were laughing, whereas me, I'd narrowly missed having my fucking head blown off. Shit. But it gave me an idea. I stopped and said to one of the Power men:
"Could I have a balloon, please? Not blown up."
"Of course, bruvver, we got hundreds. You wanna hear more about the Power of Jesus? Come and – "
"Not now, mate. Just the balloon. Please."
He gave me three limp flat balloons and laid his hand on my shoulder, strong.
"The Power of Jesus, bruvver. Call the number on the balloon. It's free."
"Sure."
Day of Power, mate, no kid.

At least my target made it easy. He was walking up the hill on the other side, didn't see me. Dr Ian Trogg, in jeans and a red T shirt, looking younger than his Next sale gear usually did. I tracked him.

This is what he did.

Went into a newsagents and came out with The Mirror, stood and studied the back pages, then Ladbrokes where he took hours picking losers, then Costcutters for a pint of milk. Boring, but I watched him closely, edgy and desperate. No more shopping please. I badly wanted him to go back to the flat so I could get on with it. And he did.

I waited a couple of minutes, then rang the bell. When he opened the door, I did a nice smile and hi! and he pretended to be pleased to see me and said,
"Er, Alex! come in. Want a coffee?"

"I've been left in charge," he said, like it was a big responsibility living for free in Karen's flat.
"Karen said you might like some company while she's away."
"Very thoughtful of her," he lied.
He went into the kitchen to make his breakfast and I sat in the lounge with the purple wall and the life-size pink and red nude by Matisse or a friend of Celia's, who cares? I was thinking about the last time I was here, having sex with Karen.
"How's that mate of yours? Mc, Mc - " Ian was calling from the kitchen.
"McEwan. He's in Rome."
He stood in the doorway beaming.

"Rome eh? Nice one! Friday night at the Forum!" He posed for his Julius Caesar act, with dramatic hands and big voice. "Friends, Romans, countrymen, I speak to you today about the evil of the Hamburger Empire. Also known as MacDonalds. Do not eat them. We will defeat them." He cracked up at his own joke. "Hahaha. He'll be good in Rome, him. He's a good laugh, isn't he?"

"Mmm," I said, meaning fuck off, he's my mate not yours.

He'd always preferred McEwan to me, even if he couldn't remember his name. He gave me a coffee which I didn't drink and he sat down on the massive red sofa with a stack of toast and coffee.

"Toast, Alex?"

"No ta."

He took a mouthful and looked at me, a touch suspicious.

"So how's young Alex?

So I tell him. I tell him how bored I am, on me summer hols in Streatham Hill, and how I remember his story about playing the dice game and the dice telling him to rob a launderette and seduce the physics teacher's wife and such kak. He chuckles in his toast. Now he's gonna believe me and <u>my</u> kak.

"So basically I've been doing the dice game myself," I tell him, "You know, to relieve the boredom."

"Oh yeah?" he says, and his eyes get curious and sharper.

"Anyway, to cut a long story short," I ramble on, "I decided to raise the stakes and take some chances. To be honest, Ian, I'd played on the safe side. So I loaded some tough options, right? Result was - the dice told me to get a gun and carry it around for a week."

He sits up, chews his toast slower. I carry on like it's no big deal.

"So I went and borrowed a neat little Colt 25 from a kid at college who collects them. He's repeating his GCSEs."

"Yeah?" He's impressed, doesn't finish his toast.

"Then my next throw of course had to be – what do I do with the gun?"

"Don't tell me – a massacre in Brixton market," he says, hopeful.

I ignore that. I tell him the options I put on the dice.

"Scare the neighbours' cat, scare the neighbours, see off a street robber, give me mum a nervous breakdown, or come and see you. Nothing violent and unpleasant, of course."

"Of course not."

"And guess what."

"Here you are." He's gone serious.

"Here I am."

He studies me, thinking hard. He's worried now alright.

"But why me, Alex?" he says quietly. "What have I got to do with it?"

"I don't like you living off Karen."

He raises his eyebrows, surprised.

"Really?"

"Yeah, what are you doing here?" I sound hard.

"I'm just staying in her flat, man. My wife's kicked me out and I need somewhere to kip. Karen said come and live here. She wants me here, right?" Then he screwed up his face, narked. "What's it got to do with you anyway? I know you fancy her but - "

"She was with _me_ - till you moved in." Not sure how to put it. "She was sick of you."

He chokes up a sarcastic laugh.

"Did she tell you that?" He pulls a mocking face and sits forward on the edge of the sofa, puts his hands out to me, quite confident, like he knows what's going on. "Hey, Alex. This is all crap, isn't it? Like your gun."

So I pull out the gun and hold it, flat on my hand. He's a long way across the room. He stares at it, gobsmacked, not at all sure what to do.

"Bloody hell, man. That's a…a replica, isn't it?" It's obvious he doesn't know and I feel in control, powerful.

"The boy I got this from doesn't do fakes and mishapes, mate. He's for real." I click the catch to make it sound real, real and lethal. He jumps.

"Not loaded though, is it?"

I nod.

"Sorry, mate."

"Show me."

I'm thinking about opening the cartridge thing and waving at him cos he won't know the difference, then I think again and smile at him, seeing his game. He'd rush me, wouldn't he?

"You'll just have to believe me, Ian."

I look him straight in the eye. He doesn't know if he believes me. We go silent for a minute. I watch him weighing up the situation. This is where he feels the pain, the panic, my revenge. This is what I'm here for. It's going well. Then he says:

"So what are you going to do, Alex? Shoot me? Seriously? You gone mad? This is a joke, isn't it?"

I blank him and he continues. He's getting narked.

"But of course - I'm forgetting, aren't I? This is Brixton. Brixton fucking gangsta town. It's how you do business here, isn't it? I don't how you stick it. There's always someone in your face, screaming at you, pushing you, psyching you out. Now you. You think this is cool don't you? Some kind of act to make you feel big. You're crazy. This isn't about me and Karen.... Are you a crack head or something? You are, aren't you? You want money? I've got £50 cash."

"No thanks."

"You're not a crack head?"

I shake my head. He's losing it. He says:

"Come on then, big boy, get it over with."

He spreads his arms and hands out, daring me, testing me, taking the piss. He freezes like that, annoying me. I laugh, sort of. Fuck him. Fuck his Brixton gangsta town. He just hates Brixton. And anyway, mate, I'm not a Brixton bad boy, me, I'm a smart-arse A-level student from Streatham, remember?

"Alex. You've got a gun in your hand. Put it down, man."

He sounds strong and sensible suddenly. But I've still got my plan, my mad plan, and I can't stop now. I keep hold of the gun and keep watching him. Then he starts to talk personal.

"OK Alex. You hate me because I'm with Karen, right? You think I'm some smooth operator who picks up young women and messes them up. Listen, let me tell you a few things about me. My marriage has fallen apart, man, I can't get to see my children, and I hardly have the money to feed myself. Karen has been an angel to me. I coulda killed myself without her. I love my kids, man."

He's looking down, rubbing his thighs. When he looks up, there are tears in his eyes. I don't want this.

"I'm not the smart arse academic you think I am, man. The job down here's finished and all I've got are a few hours at Merseyside Uni and that's it. That's why I'm trying to write this bloody text-book. I'm desperate. And Karen has saved me. So, Alex, man, if this is a joke, OK you've had your laugh, now piss off. If it's not, listen to me. This is no solution. It will only make things worse. Put the gun down and go home. Alex."

He's pulling a desperate face, worrying me. I hate that. But I still know he's a lying bastard.

"You hurt Karen. That's why she dumped you."

"What?"

"I saw the cut. Behind her ear. Where you hit her."

He shrugs, shakes his head, like he doesn't know what I'm on about. I don't trust him. He could do something silly. It's time to change the action. I lift up the Colt and point it at my head. I look straight at him and I tell him:

"I never said I was going to blast <u>you</u>, did I? I haven't told you what the dice actually landed on. Listen. It said: be a martyr to love, eliminate myself, snuff it in other words in front of my rival, which is you. Pretty exciting throw that one, Ian. I mean, fuckinell mate. I wanted it to be you or the cats who got it, but it had to land on <u>me</u>, didn't it? Poor little Alex. Tragic."

I manage a smile. I feel better threatening to kill myself. I've got more control. I watch the look in Ian's eyes shift from fear of a violent death, to relief about staying alive, then to panic at a boy suicide in his lounge, and rage at being conned, probably. He takes a chance, he knows it's all kak really, but still ain't sure. He says:

"How can you do this to me, Alex? Look, stop the bullshitting and give me the gun. I know it's a fake."

He starts to get up. He thinks it's all over. I jerk the Colt at my head and flick the catch again and he decides to sit back down to avoid boy brains suddenly hitting the polished wood floor. I tell him:

"You see, it all fits really, doesn't it? I wanted Karen. I lose Karen. I've had my chances. I've lived life to the full. I did it my way. So please don't try to stop me, Ian. Cos this is fucking fate, mate. It's the dice, innit?"

He stares at me. I wanna bring this to an end, I've had enough. He says:

"Alex, fuck the dice. This is real life. I don't know what you think you're doing but you're just a kid, man. Karen thinks you're great. You're young. You've got it all to live for."

I have to laugh, not sure I can take this.

"What about your parents?" he says.

"Me Dad's dead and me Mum needs more space."

"Alex, she'd be devastated. You know she would."

I've had enough. Enough of him pleading with me to stay alive. I've made my point, I've just gotta finish it off properly. I get up and walk across the room to the door, still holding the Colt tight and close. Ian watches, unsure of me. Closer up, I see how much he's sweating. At the door I tell him:

"Er, thanks for the encouragement."

As I walk out the door, he says:

"Alex. Leave the gun here, for God's sake." In his daddy voice again.

I pause in the doorway.

"Bye Ian. Please don't follow me."

I go downstairs and open the front door. I put the gun away and pull an orange balloon out. I listen for Ian following me – nothing. I blow the balloon up fast and DAY OF POWER gets bigger and bigger and then BANG! I smash it loud and clear. Yes! Ian starts clattering down the stairs, I slam the door and leg it. When I grab a look back I see Ian Trogg, a blob in the middle of the road, waving and mouthing at me. He wants to kill me, hurt me, scar me. No chance mate. I stagger up Brixton Hill into the clouds over Streatham High Road. I know where I'm going, but he doesn't.

I fall on my bed, exhausted and tense. I've shown the pig. Made him sweat, made him squeal. My day of power alright. But there's noone to tell, is there? Noone to laugh at my sick joke. McEwan's the only one who'd get it. And he's out of it.

I don't know what music I want and the radio's crap. I crash my CD's onto the floor and kick them. I don't get it - revenge should be sweet and I feel like shit. I flick on the telly. They're crashing fucking jets into New York and people are running for their lives. I can't stop watching it. This is real. I think about Karen and McEwan out there in the world, on aeroplanes, in strange cities, on their own.

When me Mum gets home she's terrified. She keeps looking out the window up at the sky and seeing terrorists hijacking planes left right and centre.
"You're not going out tonight, are you, Alex?" she says, dead serious.
"Nowhere special."
"You just don't know what might happen, love. They could hit London next."
"But not Streatham Hill, Mum."
She's not laughing. You can see Canary Wharf quite big from Brixton Hill. She says:
"Stay in, love. Please."
So I stay in to keep her company, watching the TV horrorshow of the rape and slaughter of the twin towers. People jumping a hundred floors to escape death in the office. Mum keeps closing her eyes and groaning, then she says,
"I can't stand this. Let's go to a pub."

The Horse and Groom was quiet, all 19 TV screens blank, out of respect, just the pulse of bass chillout songs from the system and the clash of pool balls. We sat on a bright red sofa, me Mum and me, at the heart of Streatham's multi-coloured premier sports bar. She said:

"This is such a nightmare, Alex. You know, you can handle your own bad times, you try to work things out, you do your best, don't you, but this is so mad, so hopeless."

She held her hands out, appealing to the sense and goodness of everyone in the Horse and Groom and the whole wide world.

"What I hate is - there's these terrifying men who think they've got some God-given message to kill ordinary people for. It's always bloody men. And God."

She was looking at me, teardrops in her eyes. I wanted to help, say something big, something meaningful in return, but I couldn't think straight. I was getting flashes of me and Ian and my Colt 25, shots of fear and shame. Then me Mum sighs deep and says, to lighten the mood:

"Looking forward to Karen coming home, love?"

"Nah. We're finished," I announce, quiet and definite.

I'm shocked. I've just killed off Karen. I had to, didn't I? It was obvious. I can't go back there. Me and Karen are dead. Me Mum stares at me, searching for cracks, and I stare back, very clear, then she says:

"OK, love."

And that was that.

And that was my day of power basically. My stab at Brixton gun terror. What the hell would she say, me Mum, if I told her about her little Alex's violent lover's revenge, eh?

"So proud," she'd say. "Just like your dad. Proud and bloody stupid. Now give me the gun, you silly, silly boy."

I must've been looking at her strange, cos she smiled like she knew, and put her hand on mine.

"Wanna cigarette?" I said.

And she took one, even though she doesn't smoke any more. That made us both feel better.

A BITTA PEACE AN QUIET

The dust settled and the leaves fell. A new year at Lambeth College. I studied hard and stayed quiet, let nothing disturb me.

"You've changed, Alex," said me Mum, trying to work out the difference. "You're gentler. Not so moody. Not so proud."

Boring is what she meant. A-level zombie-boy. Not coming home at dawn, cold and confused, any more. After McEwan, after Karen and all the kicks and passion, I was cooling off, getting sorted, facing facts.

Course, me Mum worried more than ever now. About the tubes and buses, Bush and the bombers, the deadly men. She was dead scared they'd strike again, sore and proud and mad. No humility, no respect. Like me, like most people, she just wanted a bitta peace and quiet.

I made a new friend. Amna. She was at college all along but I never took no notice till she cut her long black hair short, looked cool suddenly and started talking in class. She was smart and neat, dark and deep. And I was interested. We talked, in the café, on the common, on the streets. Just friends.

I applied to universities to do film courses. Film with photography, film with philosophy, film with phuck-all. I went to the movies a lot, Amna didn't do clubs, couldn't be home late. So we sat up close in The Ritzy watching Chinese gangstas and crunching popcorn. Sweet.

When Karen called, full of Morocco, I wasn't rude and I wasn't matey. She told me Ian had scarpered, quit Brixton: did you see him? Just once, I said. What did he say? She was searching. Nothing much, I said. How was he? Sweaty, I said. But I didn't tell her about my day of power, didn't say anything much cos I didn't want her to make me sad so I stayed hard, and it worked, kind of. Except I coulda strangled her.

One November night, Lizzie McEwan screamed at me across the wall of sound of a Clapham bar where she was doing some serious under-age bingeing.

"Paul's in Spain now," she bawled in my ear, kissing me, shoving me, showing off her new fun friends. "Barcelona."

"What's he doing there?" I shouted back politely, not giving a toss.

"Dunno. He sends me some very freaky messages. He thinks you hate him. You don't, do you?"

"Nah."

"He might come home for Christmas. He wants to see you."

"Yeah?"

But I didn't want to see him, did I? Didn't want him making me mad again. We'd gone our own ways. Split. And I'd changed. Nowamin?

When I told Amna I was edgy about McEwan coming home, I got narked cos she didn't understand how me and him could ever of been bruvvers. He'd called her a black angel once at college, stood too close up and rude, and she hated him. But I was different. I gave her respect. So how could you and him be best mates? she said, looking deep into my eyes. You jealous? I said, and she said no! then sulked. Poor Amna. She wanted to read my heart, but she couldn't. Trouble was, nor could I.

HOME 4 XMAS

The text from McEwan said:
"Home 4 xmas c u."
I felt sick, didn't reply.

Then Lizzie called, in a right state.
"You've got to see him, Alex, he's not well."
"What do you mean?"
"He's a wreck. And it's all <u>so</u> horrible, Alex. Mum's been screaming at him since Gatwick cos he's so skinny and ill and he's got no clothes and Dad's telling her to shut up and be happy cos Paul's home and it's Christmas, and Paul's saying crazy things like Christmas is for dogs and he can't possibly stay with us. He's just come home, for God's sake. Please see him, Alex, make him feel at home."
"Thanks alot," I said.
"Oh please," she said. "Please help."

I did not feel like helping. He didn't help me with my troubles, did he? And his family fuck-ups made me nervous. But – how can I refuse Lizzie? And, well, he's still a mate, kind of, and now he's a mate in a state. So I call him.
"Welcome home, mate!" I shout warmly like old pals.
"Yeah," he says, like he's forgotten how to talk.
Meet up? Yeah. Today, now? Yeah. Café on the common. He can't do pubs cos he's got no money. No Euros, no clothes, no nuffin.

On the bus I'm seeing ghosts. Danger signs from the past. The stupid stunts, the lies, the agony and ecstasy. McEwan. And now he's back in Streatham and I'm on my way to meet him. But I can't get things clear, can't see through the foggy, scratched-up bus window. I don't want to see him. I watch the blurry Christmas lights on the High Road flashing past, then suddenly I'm on the common and walking up the hill, blowing clouds of steam. I feel a sickly sense of responsibility.

He's standing outside the café. It's freezing cold up there and he's only got his thin grey hoodie, too small and tight, hood on, hands in. And I'm in like a big woolly jumper, thick bomber jacket, scarf and hat, and I'm still fucking shivering and stamping.

He's pale and thin, bits of wispy red beard round his chin, orrible business. We strike hands and he looks away, nervous, and I don't know what to say. He's not mouthing off and joking me like he should be.
"Got a fag, mate?"
I give him one and light it. Sucking in the flame he looks old and bony in its shadows. He draws in deep and smiles. Something's happened to his teeth, like he's lost some. He's had a rough time.

The café's almost empty. Two hot chocolates, please. We sit down, chairs scraping loud.

"Well," I say. "How's it been?"

He sips his chocolate and chews his cheeks, then tells me slowly and quietly his terrible tale of love. How he'd met the most beautiful girl in Rome and they had fallen hopelessly, madly, deeply in love. When she left for Barcelona where she studied, he couldn't live without her so he went to Spain to find her. And when he found her, guess what, she was with the Barca boy she hadn't told him about and who, it turned out, didn't want McEwan around. He never saw her again. And there he was, bust and alone in Barcelona, living in squats with pigs who ripped him off, did him over and dropped him in shit. So he left town and drifted, broken-hearted, relying on kindness. He's been sick, hungry and he's got no clothes. He pauses, holds out his hands, shrugs:

"But who needs clothes?"

"Me, for example."

I'm listening hard. It's a tragic tale, and I believe him. He had tears in his eyes for the first time ever. Love really hurts. I get us more chocolate.

And he keeps talking. His top story is the bull-run in a bored hilltop town where they block off the streets and let gangs of bulls loose on the locals: suicidal studs and sad dads who like kiss-chase with wild beasts. He, of course, having nothing to lose, can't resist the risk, jumps the fence and runs like shit. And runs and runs. Then trips and gets gored in the back by a fucking bull.

"Yer what?" I scream, not believing.

So he pulls up his tee shirt and shows me a scar on his back, proud, bruised and red. But a bull hole? Fuck knows.

"Extreme experience, Alex," he says, eyes shining now. "Very close."

"Fuck that, mate." I can't look at it, always hated body-piercing, it's sick. Like his cuts and burns. And now he's showing it off to the sweet Italian café mamma who's taking a big interest. He's making pointy bull horns with his hands to explain. She gasps.

I sit him down to protect him. He waggles his horns and grins at me. I point at his teeth, not all there.

"So what happened to the er teeth?"

"Village brawls. You know. Spanish cowboys." He smiles, embarrassed, then covers his mouth. "Fucking sore, mate."

He sucks the gaps in, blows them out. In, out, in, out. I'm staring at him. He's not just mad any more, he needs rescuing and feeding and a new fucking family. He knows I'm vexing about him. He says quietly:

"Can I come back to your place, mate? I can't go home. I – "

"Sure, mate." He didn't need to explain. "Me Mum's there. She'd love to see you."

She better had.

"I like your mum," he says. "Has she forgiven me for everything?"

"Everything."

He chuckles, relieved.

On the bus, he stares out at the High Road lights, the Christmas junk, Odeon, Caesars. He's sucking in and blowing out, and I'm thinking people must be looking at him, knowing he's troubled, but they're not looking, they don't even notice, cos people's got their own troubles on busses.

I call me Mum to warn her I'm bringing my old mate McEwan home for tea. Don't worry, she says, I know all about it, I've had his mum on the phone for an hour.

Walking up the road, I want to ask him about the overdose he never told me about, but I don't, it's too edgy and I don't believe it anyway. So I just say:
"What's it like coming home then?"
He thinks about it.
"I'm done in, mate. Haven't slept for weeks. I had to come back. Nowamin?"
"Yeah."

He asks about me and Karen and I say:
"Finished, mate. Dead. Ended."
"Anyone else?"
"Nah," I lied. "Not worth it, is it?"
Girls are bad news basically and I want to keep Amna out of this.
"Fucking women," he says with feeling and fists a neighbour's hedge.
We go quiet, thinking about fucking women. I'm thinking: funny how you don't stay mates with girls

when you finish, but you can still be mates with mad bastards like McEwan. Innit?

I'm home, with McEwan. Shit, what happens now?

Well, he adores Mum's Christmas tree for a start and makes her smile. It's the old charm and gush. Then he says to her:
"Mrs Alex, I want to apologise for messing up at that party for your sad kids."
"Paul, it's a long time ago now, but thank you."
She gives his bony body a hug and me a wink at the same time. She knows I'm relying on her.

When he's in the bog we talk in whispers.
"How is he?" she asks.
"Wrecked."
"His mum's so upset. They had no idea. He just called them from Spain and said fly me home. His dad's going to take him to the doctor in the morning.
He – "
He comes in sucking his cheeks, thoughtful, hood off at last, new dreads tangled and flat. He stands in the middle of the room and says, looking at nothing:
"Do you think…Can I stay here tonight, please?"
"Yes, Paul. I've already talked with your mother and told her that's fine."
"Thanks," he says, frowning. "What's she saying, my Mum?"
"Well, she knows you need time to adjust to being home again. And she's concerned about your

health, Paul. Your dad's going to take you to the doctor's in the morning."

"Really not necessary," he mutters. He's stranded in the middle of the room, like a refugee.

"Sit down, Paul," me Mum says. "You must be exhausted after all your wild adventures."

He nods, closes his eyes and collapses on the floor, mouth wide open, teeth missing. Resting. Then he smiles at her, the old mischievous look. She says:

"I'll make up the sofabed."

"Thanks, Mrs Alex."

"Call me Pat, remember."

"Pat. Pat..."

He could hardly talk any more, scratching his head to make sense, sitting there, middle of nowhere. Then he holds up his hand and says:

"Sorry. Something to tell you." Pause, a little smile.

"The wife and the donkey are waiting outside."

It took us a minute, then we roared. Christmas.

HELP

McEwan shouted out loud in his sleep.

"Who were you shouting at, Paul?" me Mum asks him at breakfast.

"My mum probably. Or Bush. Or God," he says. "Someone who needs a good ear-bashing."

I'm trying not to look at him cos he looks so white and wasted in daylight. Mum's waiting for the toast, wondering what would help the troubled boy. She has a suggestion.

"Do you ever listen to your own voice, Paul? Try being quiet sometimes and just listening. It might tell you what you're needing."

She could be so Zen and Yoga sometimes.

"Problem is I mainly talk crap, Pat."

Mum smiles but she's serious.

"Try it some time," she says.

So he does, there and then, hands over ears, staring into the deep of his tea and listening for his inner voice. Silence. When he surfaces, eyes closed, he proclaims like a holy man:

"Little voice say: only go to doctor if Alex come too."

"OK, mate," I say.

His dad arrives, tense, thanks me Mum for looking after his big boy.

"Why am I seeing this doctor?" McEwan asks him.

"You're not looking well, Paul, and everyone's concerned about you. Let's just see what the doctor says."

"I want Alex to come," says McEwan, grabbing my arm.

"No problem, no problem at all," his dad says, anything to get him to the doctor.

"I mean I want him to come in with me. But not you."

"OK, Paul." Rejected Dad nods and tries to smile at me Mum.

In the car he asks me about my future plans and I say Hollywood or Streatham Odeon. McEwan's giggling in the backseat, sucking his cheeks in and out. Mr McEwan's not amused.

The waiting room's crammed with old codgers and kids with colds. The receptionist only squeezes McEwan in after his dad leans across the desk and convinces her, confidentially, that his boy's an urgent case. Us three nervous wrecks stand, me in the middle, and wait.

"Why am I here?" McEwan asks me in a loud whisper, acting dumb.

"Cos you need help, mate."

"HELP! HELP!" he shouts and makes all the ill people jump.

"Paul!" says his father, ashamed and about to burst.

McEwan smiles at everyone, arms out and goes: "Sorry, guys. It's the stress. It's the NHS."

He giggles like he's 10. I want this to end. I want to go home.

"Paul McEwan. Room 3."

His dad glares at him, pokes him, and McEwan slowly moves, faking a terrible limp to the door, then pushes me in first. The doctor has trendy specs. He looks at us, not sure which one's in pain.

"I'm just his friend," I explain. "He wants me here. His dad's in there."

I point towards the waiting room, want him to know we're not alone. He nods and turns, all ears, to McEwan who explains:

"My parents have sent me here, but I'm OK really, just back from Spain, a bit sick, a bit dodgy, need a rest cos it's a dog's life, Doctor, nowamin? Oh, and my teeth."

"What about your teeth?"

"I've lost some."

The doctor shines a torch in his mouth then his eyes, and takes his pulse.

"So what were you doing in Spain, Paul?" he says, chatty-style.

"Pestering a girl and getting kicked."

"I see." The doctor checks the medical notes for clues.

"Anything that you're worrying about at the moment?"

McEwan frowns.

"I worry about the world, doctor."

"What exactly?"

"Well. The global nightmare of course."

"The global nightmare," the doctor repeats, like he's impressed.

"Exactly", says McEwan. "And my failure to prevent it."

"Mmm." The doctor's sucking his specs, thinking deep.

"What drugs do you take now, Paul?"

"Only the best Brixton skunk, doctor."

"How often?"

"Special occasions."

"I'd lay off it altogether. It can muddle your thoughts."

"Sure." McEwan nods and sticks up a thumb.

"I see you overdosed on analgesics and alcohol in April, Paul. Have you felt like doing anything like that again?"

McEwan doesn't blink or blush. He's probably forgotten he never told me about it.

"Oh no. That was dumb. I love life too much now."

I'm like jaw-dropping at this crap and his nerve. Trouble is, the doctor don't understand. He says:

"I'd like to ask your father to join us, Paul, if that's OK with you."

"Good idea, Doctor. He needs something for his stress levels."

"I want to talk to him about you. OK?"

McEwan shrugs. Doctor buzzes. Mr McEwan walks in. I curl up. Doctor says:

"Paul says you're concerned about him."

"Absolutely," says Mr McEwan, on the edge of his seat, dying to tell. "He's come home looking terrible. Just look at him. He's lost weight, lost teeth, even lost his clothes. Look, Paul's had his problems in the past, but he was always a bright, outgoing boy – till this year." Quick glance at me, the cause of it all. Your little Alex, maligned and stigmatised. Life is so unfair. Fuck off, McEwan's dad. Just fuck off. "And now he's up then he's down - mostly down - and yes we are worried. When your son's been through one suicide attempt, you don't take any chances."

McEwan reaches out to his desperate dad.

"But Dad, listen, this is different. I lost my <u>heart</u> in Barcelona, not just my clothes, right? I fell in love with a girl in Rome and she loved me too. I followed her across the sea, but she dumped me, right, and I got hurt. And I'm still mending my broken heart. Nowamin?"

McEwan's love story. He's crying again but doesn't seem to mind. I stare at the floor. His dad's speechless. The doctor clears his throat and says, matter of fact like:

"Paul, I think you need some help to get over your er distress and I want you to see a colleague from the Community Mental Health Team. Tomorrow morning, 9 o'clock, OK?"

"What no pills?" says McEwan.

"No I don't think you need pills right now. I think you need to keep talking about what's troubling you."

"Talk, not pills."

"Exactly, Paul. And a dentist."

McEwan shakes his hand.

"Thanks, Doc. Very good."

Walking to the car, Mr McEwan says, kindly:

"You didn't tell us about the girl, Paul."

"No it was too – I dunno. I've been through a lot, Dad, you know?"

His dad nods like of course he understands, man to man, father and son. But I'm thinking about his blagging, all this love of life and broken heart crap, just like he used to blag about sex and revolution. When's he going to get real?

We get in the car. I grab the back seat. McEwan says:

"Can I come back to your place, Alex?"

"Paul," his father intervenes, serious and teacher-like. "It's time to come home. Your mother and Lizzie have been longing to see you for months. We've all missed you. Stay at home for now."

"But we always argue. I'm like a war zone for you lot. I just cause you grief, don't I? "

"We'll talk, I promise, Paul. There's no need to argue."

Mr McEwan's trying hard to hold onto his sick boy and keep him safe. I don't like him; he thinks I'm to blame. He says:

"Alex can come round if you like."

No thanks mate. Fuckinell. McEwan goes quiet. They're both staring at the windscreen, not looking at each other, talking like I'm not there.

"Look Paul, we need to talk, all of us, catch up on things. Lizzie's dying to hear all your adventures."

McEwan sucks his cheeks. His dad goes on pressing.

"Be at home today, Paul. You need to take care, get warm and fed. You look half-starved. Stay in today."

I cough and say I better go, got shopping to do. Christmas presents. Nowamin.

"Of course, Alex," says Mr McEwan. "Thank you for your help. And your mum. You must both come round sometime. What about New Year's Eve?"

Oh no. I get out. So does McEwan.

"Thanks mate." He gives me a hug. "We'll talk. Like the doc said."

Then he gets back in the car. I wish they'd given him the pills.

STREATHAM HIGH ROAD

Lizzie called that evening and said is he with you? They hadn't seen him since the family row at lunchtime. He was sore and he'd slammed out of the house. It was dark now and Lizzie was frightened.

"He won't answer his phone, Alex. You must call us if he shows up. You will, won't you?"

"Yeah, don't worry, he's cool."

"He's <u>not</u>, Alex. And he's got to see the doctor tomorrow morning, before Christmas."

I could hear his parents panicking beside her. His dad took over the phone, urgent. He said:

"Alex, where do you think he's likely to be? One of the pubs on the High Road?"

"Could be, but he could be anywhere." Fuck knows.

"We're worried about him, Alex. Very worried. Would you check the pubs your end of Streatham? I'll take the ones this end. From the Odeon. Is that OK?"

Bloody ell. But I had to, didn't I? McEwan was in shit and his father was desperate. We exchanged mobile numbers.

"Thank you, Alex." He sounded pissed off and polite at the same time. "And if you find him, call me and I'll come and get him."

"Er OK."

I was on my own. Me Mum was at her work's Christmas night out, getting mashed and rude. No Mum to drive me, so I've gotta run, get my boots on, get out and find the sad boy. This is mad. And it's fucking cold out there.

Then McEwan calls. The bad boy himself. Muffled sound, lots of background. I say:
"Where are you, mate?"
"The station."
"Which one?"
"Streatham. I mean, Streatham Hill."
"Where are you going, mate?"
"Nowhere."
He's slow, slurred. But I'm speeding, wanna sort it, go home and stay warm.
"You pissed up, mate?"
"Nah."
"So what are you doing?"
"Thinking."
"Lizzie's really worried about ya."
He doesn't reply. I can hear him breathing. Then he says:
"I wanna tell you something, Alex."
Pause.
"Go on, mate."
"All that about the girl in Spain was crap."
"Yeah?"
"Yeah. There was a girl but I only saw her once, man, nowamin?"
"Yeah I know."
"I tried to get close, you know, and her boyfriend thumped me in Barcelona."
He stops, so I say shit, man, to sympathise and he says:

"I was on the streets for weeks, nowhere to go. Like one of them boys with a blanket, you know, on the street, dossing and thieving. I got beaten up, cops took me to hospital, doctors kicked me out. I couldn't move so I came home."

"Fuckin ell, man." I try to lighten him up. "But what about the bull?"

"What bull?"

"The one that stuck you."

"Shoulda killed me."

"Piss off."

I have to keep him talking so I can rescue him and be a hero for Lizzie. He's got to see the doctor tomorrow to get the pills before Christmas. He says:

"I want you to know the truth, Alex. I can talk to you. But don't tell my parents, will ya? They'll kill me."

"They're just worried about you, mate. They're looking for ya, they wanna know you're alive and er kicking."

Silence. I shouldn't have told him they were looking for him. He starts quiet and serious and ends up shouting at me:

"Don't tell them where I am. Don't tell them, Alex. I want to be on my own tonight. Right? You tell em, tell em I'm alive and kicking and screaming. And I'm not seeing any more doctors. Got that? NO FUCKING DOCTORS. They do me in."

"OK, mate. You're safe."

I can hear train announcements in the background.

"You definitely at Streatham Hill, mate?"

"Yeah."

"OK. I'm coming to meet you and we can go for a beer or something, right?"

There are three stations strung along Streatham High Road. People always go to the wrong one. Streatham Hill's the nearest. I'm two minutes away and I'm walking and talking fast. It's a freezing night, frost and fog over everything, Christmas trees flashing like lighthouses.

"Cold, innit?" I yell.

"Battery's low, mate," he says, quietly.

"You or the phone?"

"Both, mate."

Course, when I get to the station, he's not there, is he? Shit. I look all over, tracks included. I ask people. Noone's seen him. Must be a different station. He's joking me. I call him again and he answers.

"Where are you mate?"

"Going somewhere quiet."

"Like where?"

"The woods."

"What woods?"

"Up the hill. You can see the moon up there."

"On your own? In the dark?"

"Yeah, and don't tell my dad, OK? OK? Promise?"

"OK."

"Thanks mate. Seeya tomorrow."

I believe him.

I call Mr McEwan:

"Paul phoned me and said he's at Streatham Hill station – "

"Thank God."

"But I'm here now and he's not. But he was definitely at a station. I could hear the trains."

"Oh God."

He's thinking Paul-under-a-train total disaster, isn't he? But I know that's crap. He's gone to the woods for the moon and a bitta peace an quiet, but I can't tell his dad that, can I? I promised.

So Mr McEwan races to Streatham Common Station where the fast trains whiz past, and I get a bus to Streatham Station near the Ice Rink. I keep phoning McEwan but he doesn't answer so I leave a message: call me. But he doesn't. I call our neighbours in the downstairs flat and ask old Mary, if a boy called Paul turns up, please take him in, he's er very cold. Course we will, darlin, we'll look after him for ya.

When I get to Streatham Station, Mr McEwan's already done Streatham Common and is standing there with two cops from the High Road beat, beaming yellow, radios buzzing with Christmas crime. Not much they can do in the circumstances, they say, but they'll look out for a tall thin white boy in a grey hoodie with TAWT on the back. Mr McEwan's expecting more of a response to find his sick boy, but the cops have more urgent calls. Thanks, he says, abandoned dad.

Mr McEwan and I stand by the screaming High Road, breathing fog and steam. He's twisting his leather gloves and straining his brain.

"Look, how did Paul sound, Alex? What exactly did he say to you?"

"Just that he was er thinking about things. I think he wants to be on his own for a while. And he's worried about seeing the doctor tomorrow."

Mr McEwan closes his eyes and goes stiff, fists clenched. He's convinced that his son is going to do something stupid tonight if we don't find him. I don't think so. He's lost but he'll come back.

"He's got to be somewhere on this damn road," his dad says, betting everything that his sick son won't stray far from the axis of evenings, the long road between Streatham and Brixton. "Will you help me, Alex?"

What I reckon is this. If McEwan needs to go to the woods for some peace and quiet, that's OK. If I tell his dad, he'll search all the woods in Streatham and there's only Streatham Common and if he finds him, it'll do McEwan's head in and I did promise didn't I? But if I search the High Road with his dad, waste of time sure, but at least I've helped, we can all go home, and McEwan walks in later, home and peaceful and chilled. And if he's lying about the woods, what the fuck can we do anyway?

So I say: yes, I'll help you, Mr McEwan, but I don't mention the woods, cos McEwan's gonna be alright, ain't he?

His phone rings a twinkley tune and he stops the car. I can hear Mrs McEwan shouting, desperate to know what's happened. He tries to calm her down, ends the call and says quietly but so I could hear.

"I wish Paul would consider other people's feelings for a change."

Bottom of Brixton Hill, my concentration wanders, I'm checking out a group of girls pissing about at a bustop.

"Concentrate, for God's sake, Alex."

He shouts at me, makes me jump, then he goes silent, peering through the mist and lights as he drives slowly back up the hill. Someone hoots and flashes him. He hisses piss off between his teeth. He's gripping the wheel tight with both hands and moans loud and angry:

"Why does my son do this to me?"

I think I know the answer cos basically I don't like McEwan's dad and he's never liked me, being a bad influence. I gotta tell him:

"He's a good boy, Mr McEwan. Give him a chance. Trust him. He'll be alright."

He says nothing.

When he stops at the lights at the Crown and Sceptre, near my home, I get out saying I'll check it out, we used to drink here. He leans across the

front seat, grabs my arm and fixes me with his eyes like McEwan did, and says:
"Paul means everything to me, Alex." He's blinking back the tears. "Like you and your dad, I'm sure."
"Yeah," I said. "Shame he's dead."

Home on me own, I want me Mum. I leave another message on McEwan's phone: call me, Paul. But he doesn't. He's in the woods.

．．．．．．．．．．．．

In the morning a friend of the McEwans called and wanted to talk to me Mum. I gave her the phone and I watched her listening, just listening, then she looked at me and closed her eyes and said: oh Alex.

At the top of the common, by the woods, there's a small playground behind a hedge, not far from the road and the roar, just two swings and an old see-saw. McEwan was found bleeding and frozen, dead under a swing.

Lizzie wanted to talk, but I couldn't. I didn't want to know it was true.

THE WOODS

Some people think McEwan killed himself, but I don't. Nobody knows what he told me that night. He went to the woods for some peace an quiet, like he said, didn't he, and I believed him. But then some twisted bastard jumped him and stuck him and left him to bleed away in the freezing dark playground. Things happen in the woods, don't they? Like the yellow warning signs said: vicious attacks and violent robberies. Not a good place.

Me Mum says we don't know the full story. She says why the hell did he go there anyway? Everyone knows those woods are dodgy at night. Perhaps he wanted to be alone, I tell her. To think straight. I never told her I knew. Do you think he was looking for men? she said, curious, cos of the woods having a reputation. What? McEwan? Men? No, Mum.

I've stuck that card he gave me, of his face on an Indian god with too many arms, on my wall with some tinsel round it and a candle underneath.
"That's nice, darling," me Mum says to be kind.
She doesn't need to, it's a joke really but she can't see it. It's Christmas, Mum.

A good boy, McEwan, wasn't he? OK he was a blagger and a liar, a mad bastard really, but he shouted about the world and evil and crap, didn't he, and he was my mate. Then he gets knifed, when he's knackered, alone in the dark woods.

Fucking luck. Eighteen years old. 2001. Start of the millennium. The year of good and evil. And now it's McEwan's. Nowamin?

Amna wants to comfort me. God is always close, she says. So why didn't he save McEwan? Perhaps He did, she says. You what, Amna? I can't talk to her, don't see it lasting. She didn't know him. Noone knew him like I did. Even his parents thought he was bad – and I'm responsible. Fuck off. He was a good boy. <u>You</u> know that, doncha? Now Lizzie thinks I've gone weird about him just cos I asked her for some of his rap and R&B and his purple hat with the ear flaps for the cold. I don't care if it's crap.

I'm wearing it tonight and I'm going out to get well and truly shucked. For McEwan. You see, mate, I don't want no grief, I wanna keep rolling. You understand, doncha? So I'm going out, mate, not sure where, but I'm rolling, rolling down the hill to Brixton, to the screaming, flashing town, sirens going, fire police ambulance, the lot, mate. I want beer with a kick and a bar with beat. There's Kids I Know at The Living Room. XRex at Dogstar. Funkt at Mass. What do you think?

Printed in the United Kingdom
by Lightning Source UK Ltd.
119239UK00001B/85-126